M. Samii M. Ammirati

Surgery of Skull Base Meningiomas

With a Chapter on Pathology by G. F. Walter

With 120 Figures in 246 Separate Illustrations, 3 in Color

Springer-Verlag
Berlin Heidelberg NewYork
London Paris Tokyo
HongKong Barcelona
Budapest

Professor Dr. med. MADJID SAMII
Medizinische Hochschule Hannover
Direktor der Neurochirurgischen Klinik am Krankenhaus Nordstadt
der Landeshauptstadt Hannover, Haltenhoffstraße 41,
W-3000 Hannover 1, FRG

MARIO AMMIRATI, M. D.
Assistant Professor, Division of Neurosurgery
University of California, Los Angeles,
Chief, Division of Neurosurgery
Olive View/UCLA Medical Center
10833 Le Conte Avenue, Los Angeles, CA 90024-6901, USA

Professor Dr. med. Dr. phil. GERHARD F. WALTER
Medizinische Hochschule Hannover
Abteilung für Neuropathologie, Konstanty-Gutschow-Straße 8
W-3000 Hannover 61, FRG

ISBN 3-540-54016-4 Springer-Verlag Berlin Heidelberg New York Tokyo
ISBN 0-387-54016-4 Springer-Verlag New York Berlin Heidelberg Tokyo
ISBN 4-431-54016-4 Springer-Verlag Tokyo Berlin Heidelberg New York

Library of Congress Cataloging-in-Publication Data. Samii, Madjid. Surgery of skull base meningiomas / M. Samii, M. Ammirati; with a chapter on pathology by G. F. Walter. p. cm. Includes bibliographical references and index. ISBN 3-540-54016-4 (alk. paper). – ISBN 0-387-54016-4 (alk. paper). 1. Meningioma – Surgery. I. Ammirati, M. (Mario) II. Walter, G. F. (Gerhard F.) III. Title. [DNLM: 1. Meningioma – surgery. 2. Skull Neoplasms – surgery. WE 707 S188s] RD593.S334 1991 616.99'281 – dc20 DNLM/DLC

Reproduction of the figures: Gustav Dreher GmbH, Stuttgart
Typesetting: K+V Fotosatz GmbH, Beerfelden
Printing: Appl, Wemding
Binding: J. Schäffer GmbH & Co. KG, Grünstadt
25/3130-5 4 3 2 1 0 – Printed on acid-free paper

Preface

Although surgery of the skull base still represents a frontier involving different specialties, it is increasingly being accepted and recognized as a special area posing both unique diagnostic and surgical challenges and specific requirements. This is the prime reason that colleagues involved in the management of skull base processes need special training stressing the different surgical approaches required either at different times or to reach the different areas of this intriguing anatomical landmark.

Although the advent of microsurgical techniques and advanced diagnostic modalities – high-resolution computed tomography, magnetic resonance imaging (MRI) and MR-angiography, and superselective endovascular protocols – in the last 25 years has brought significant improvements, such as the recent advances in endovascular treatment, a number of different kinds of limitations still persist. This is especially so in the case of skull base meningiomas, the pathological entity most frequently affecting this area which the neurosurgeon is confronted with in daily practice. Besides understanding the intrinsic characteristics of the different pathological entities which involve the skull base, it is the responsibility of physicians to know and employ the expanded neurosurgical options in the most effective and appropriate way.

This book represents a modest contribution on the subject of skull base meningiomas based on our personal experience in skull base surgery, amounting to over one thousand procedures. We have evaluated 217 meningiomas affecting the skull base, operated on in the period between January 1978 and December 1988. The philosophy for determining the most appropriate treatment, surgical techniques and options for the individual approaches are discussed separately and demonstrated by means of case presentations. We place particular emphasis on the landmarks of surgery. A further main theme is the possible complications or risks and how to avoid them by using sound anatomical-surgical criteria and proper surgical timing or decision-making.

Our book should thus be of practical value to the neurosurgeon. In addition, however, the chapter on neuropathology exposes the reader to important fundamental features, such as anatomical and biological properties, incidence, classification, and immunology that are of value in understanding these tumors and are essential knowledge when considering surgical strategy. One should not underestimate the importance of the biological behavior of meningiomas, as this is a dominant influence on surgical outcome. The boundary between benign and malignant behavior is often indistinct, as we have experienced on many occasions, and even when one considers all the data, it is still very difficult to estimate morphologically and surgically the progression of the disease in individual cases. However, basic scientists as well as neuropathologists and neuroradiologists are now approaching a new era in our understanding of the factors conditioning behavior and outcome.

Considering the importance of the topic, we felt it would be useful to report the results obtained in treating skull base meningiomas and to convey in general a specific philosophy regarding treatment of skull base tumors. Well aware of the limitations of any book, we decided to focus this volume on the crucial aspect of skull base meningiomas, providing guidelines for the microsurgical removal of pathological processes with low morbidity. In our daily work we continue to explore the problems still facing us, and hope that our book will serve as a guide and stimulus to colleagues involved in this field of neurosurgery.

Finally, we want to express our gratitude to Dr. W. Bini for his painstaking work in preparing the subject index and to Springer-Verlag and its staff for their cooperation and help in bringing this volume to print.

M. Samii
Hannover, FRG

M. Ammirati
Los Angeles, USA

Contents

CHAPTER 1

General Concepts

Meningiomas account for approximately 13%–19% of all primary intracranial neoplasms seen clinically [6, 10]. Population-based surveys on the proportion of meningiomas among all primary intracranial neoplasms report a range of 17%–23% [9, 22, 25], with a rate as high as 38.7% when autoptic data are included [12]. The estimated average annual incidence of intracranial meningiomas in the United States has been calculated at approximately 1.6 per 100 000 population [25]. Skull base meningiomas, excluding intraorbital and optic sheath tumors, accounted for 51.6% of the Mayo Clinic experience reported by McCarty and Taylor in 1979 [14]. Meningiomas are more common in women than in men, with a ratio of 2:1 for intracranial meningiomas; the peak incidence occurs at the age of 45 years [20].

On the basis of histological similarities, meningiomas are thought to arise from the cells forming the outer lining of the arachnoid membrane (arachnoidal cap cells) [10]; however, according to Rubinstein, they may occasionally originate from dural fibroblasts and pial cells [20]. If origin in the arachnoid cap cells is accepted, then the almost invariable attachment of these tumors to the dura must be regarded as a form of local invasion not dissimilar from the local invasion of other topographically related mesodermal structures, such as the skull, temporal muscle, and soft tissue of the orbit and paranasal sinuses [20]. An alternative hypothesis to explain the almost regular dural attachment of meningiomas is that of the presence of arachnoidal cell nests inside the dura, as demonstrated by Borovich [2]. Intraventricular meningiomas are explained by the presence of nests of arachnoidal cap cells associated with the choroid plexus, while the histogenesis of ectopic meningiomas is obscure, but is probably related to the presence of ectopic arachnoidal cells inclusion [13, 20].

Meningiomas are generally benign, slowly growing neoplasms. Irrespective of its surgical resectability, a practical definition of a malignant meningioma is that it is a neoplasm that invades the brain parenchyma or that gives rise to distant metastases.

The gross appearance of intracranial meningiomas is that of a globular or lobulated, firm, occasionally calcified tumor, although at times a more laminar type of growth with diffuse dural and bony invasion is seen (en plaque meningiomas). The adjacent brain is usually compressed but, other than in the rare malignant forms, is not invaded by the tumor. The dura related to the origin of the meningiomas is usually invaded, as may be other mesodermal structures related to the tumor, such as bone, temporal muscle, etc. In the en plaque meningiomas the dura and bone are diffusely invaded by the tumor, making total surgical resection more difficult. The reaction of the bone adjacent to a meningioma was extensively studied by Cushing, who described eight different patterns [6]. Suffice it to say that the bone is usually hyperostotic, and that this extensive new bone formation is not always associated with tumor invasion. Lytic skull defects usually indicate tumor invasion [16].

The relationship of meningiomas to the leptomeninges and to the subarachnoid space is dealt within Chap. 2. Numerous histological types of meningiomas have been described; Cushing listed nine major types with some 22 subvarieties [6]. Rubinstein [20] described four major types of meningiomas, namely the meningotheliomatous (endotheliomatous or syncytial), transitional, fibroblastic, and angioblastic types (Figs. 1.1–1.7). Rubinstein defined the angioblastic type on the basis of high cellularity, closely packed ovoid nuclei, and abundance of capillaries that may be dilated or compressed and hence visible only using connective tissue stains. Mitotic figures may be found while

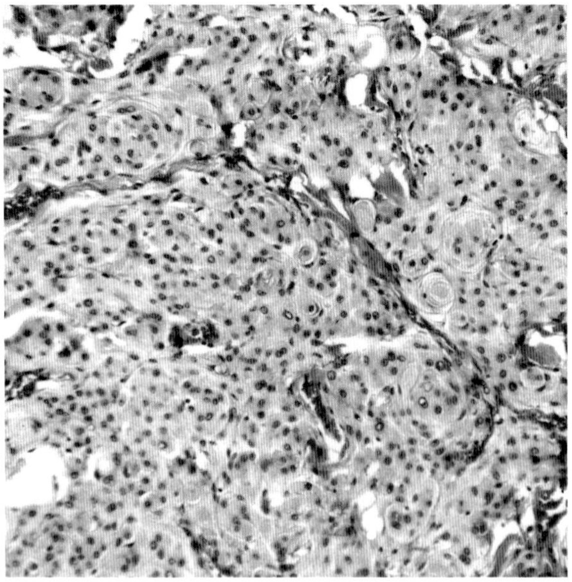

1.1

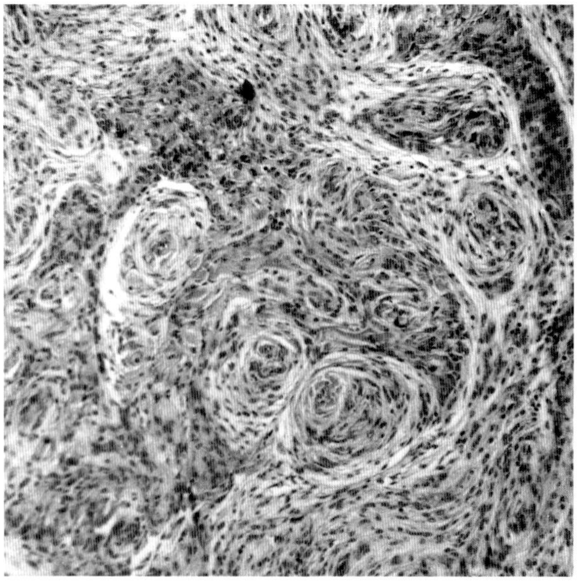

1.2

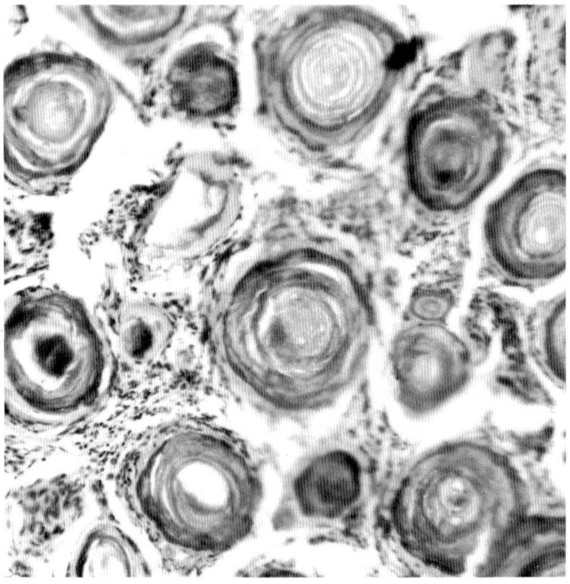

1.3

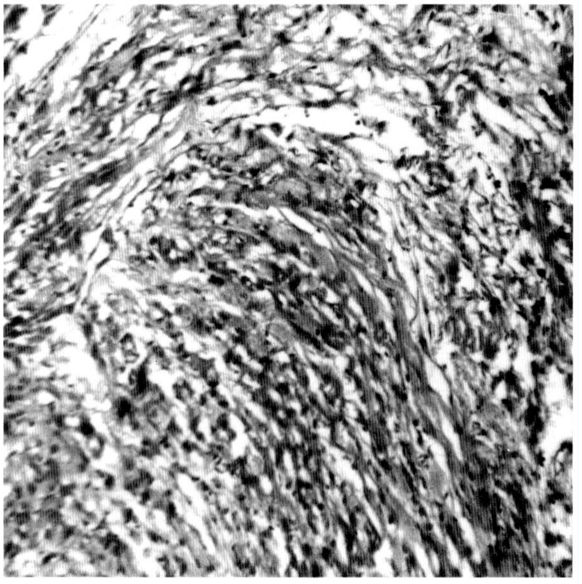

1.4

Fig. 1.1. Syncytial (meningothelial) meningioma. Sheets of meningothelial cells with indistinct borders arranged in lobules. Occasional nuclei contain "pseudoinclusion bodies" imparting an empty appearance (×300; H&E)

Fig. 1.2. Transitional meningioma. Lobular architecture composed of syncytial cells separated by fibroblastic, elongated cells. Early microwhorls suggestive of psammoma body formation (×300; H&E)

Fig. 1.3. Psammomatous meningioma. Calcific psammoma bodies are dominant, surrounded by scanty cellular elements (×300; H&E)

Fig. 1.4. Fibroblastic meningioma. Densely hyalinized and collagen-forming meningioma with nuclear elongation (×110; H&E)

1.5 a 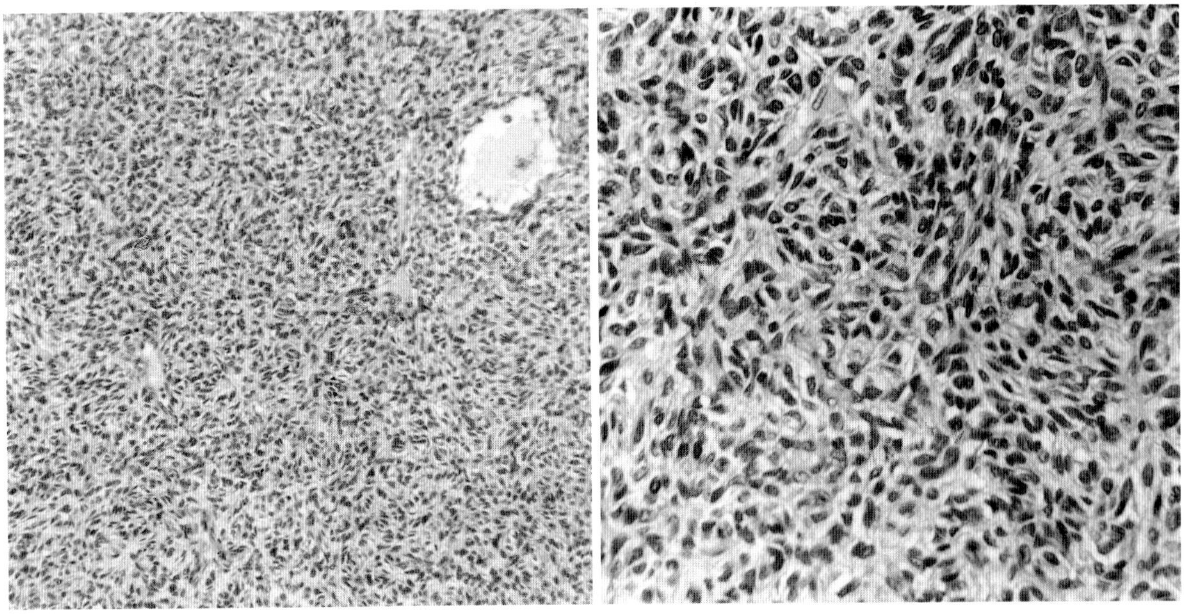 b

1.6 a 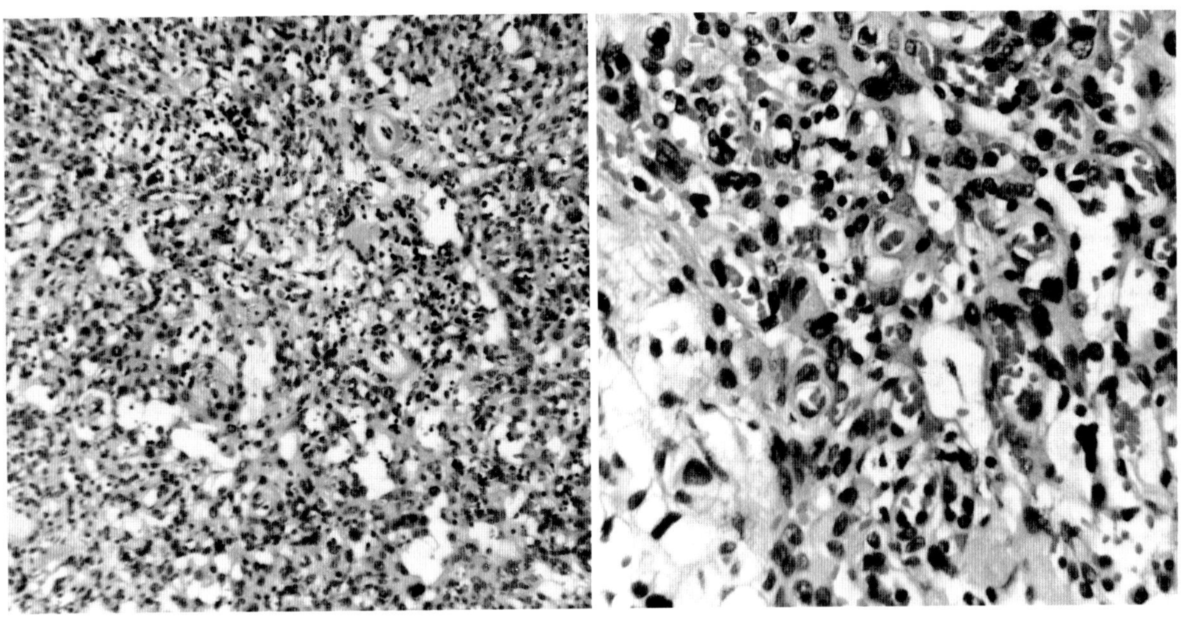 b

Fig. 1.5. **a** Angioblastic meningioma. Densely cellular, irregularly oriented, triangularly shaped nuclei. Vascular slits are not easily recognized, but reticulin stains would reveal a pericellular reticulosis (×110; H&E). **b** Angioblastic meningioma; detail of **a** (×300; H&E)

Fig. 1.6. **a** Meningeal neoplasm with numerous vascular spaces lined by endothelium; reticulin stains would outline these vascular channels (×110; H&E). **b** Detail of **a**. Note also focus of vacuoated, foamy cells (×300; H&E)

Fig. 1.1 – 1.6 with courtesy of Dr. A. Verity, Professor and Chief Neuropathology, UCLA

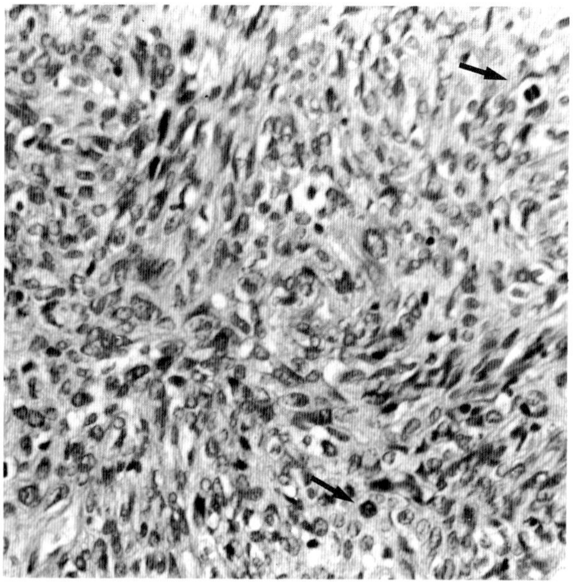

Fig. 1.7. Hypercellular meningeal neoplasm with prominent nuclear pleomorphism and rare mitoses (*arrow*) (×300; H&E)

whorls or nests of typical meningotheliomatous or transitional meningiomas are absent. The angioblastic meningioma, so defined, is histologically similar to the capillary hemangioblastoma and may indeed represent a tumor of blood space forming elements, as already suggested by Bailey [1]. This variety of meningioma is called by some hemangiopericytoma of the meninges [11]; it is most commonly located near the torcular and is perhaps more likely to develop recurrence and distant metastases than other types of meningiomas [13]. The lack of meningeal cells differentiates this tumor from the occasionally encountered highly vascular meningioma. Although the presence of atypical features such as cellular pleomorphism and mitotic figures may be worrisome (Fig. 1.7), the practical criteria that qualify a meningioma as malignant are the invasion of the brain parenchyma and the presence of distant metastases. The histological appearance of these malignant meningiomas is not necessarily atypical, and, as already pointed out, while all histological types of meningiomas may be malignant, the angioblastic variant, as defined above, seems more prone to be so [20].

The clinical presentation of skull base meningiomas is obviously related to their topographical localization; this was brilliantly described by Cushing in his monograph [6]. Meningiomas are slowly growing tumors, and in the majority of these patients it is often possible to elicit a history of headache dating back many years. Due to the noninvasive, aggressive work-up of headache and other nonspecific complaints (such as dizziness) made possible by computed tomography (CT) and magnetic resonance imaging (MRI) it is anticipated, and is partially already seen in clinical practice, that many patients harboring skull base meningiomas will be diagnosed relatively early in the course of their disease. Consequently, the clinical judgement and acumen of the neurosurgeon must shift from recognition of the "classical" syndromes of skull base meningiomas (Cushing) to the cautions exercise of judgement in recommending an operation to a patient with a relatively small meningioma, vaguely or mildly symptomatic. As the presence of meningiomas is a relatively common autoptic finding [27], and it is not possible at present to predict the growth potential of an individual tumor, it is probably wise in many such patients to choose a waiting course and to repeat the neuroradiological test in a few months to assess the eventual tumor growth. This line of action must be balanced by the fact that it is surgically easier to remove a smaller tumor.

The diagnosis of meningiomas using skull X-rays, radionuclide scan, echoencephalography, ventriculography, pneumoencephalography, and angiography belongs to the history of neurosurgery [15, 17]. Today CT is clearly the gold standard in the diagnosis of meningiomas; its sensitivity has been reported to be as high as 96% and its specificity around 90% [18]. The typical CT appearance of a meningioma is of a well-defined lesion that is moderately hyperdense in nonenhanced CT with respect to the brain parenchyma (although iso- and hypodense meningiomas are seen in 10% and 4% of cases, respectively [18]), and that enhances densely and homogeneously following contrast infusion [18] (Fig. 1.8). Nonenhanced MRI shows meningiomas poorly, while enhanced MRI shows meningiomas to a greater advantage [28] (Fig. 1.8). MRI poorly images bone, and consequently a great deal of information concerning the relationship between the tumor and the bone (erosion, hyperostosis, frank bone invasion) that is readily available with bone algorithm CT scans is lost using MRI.

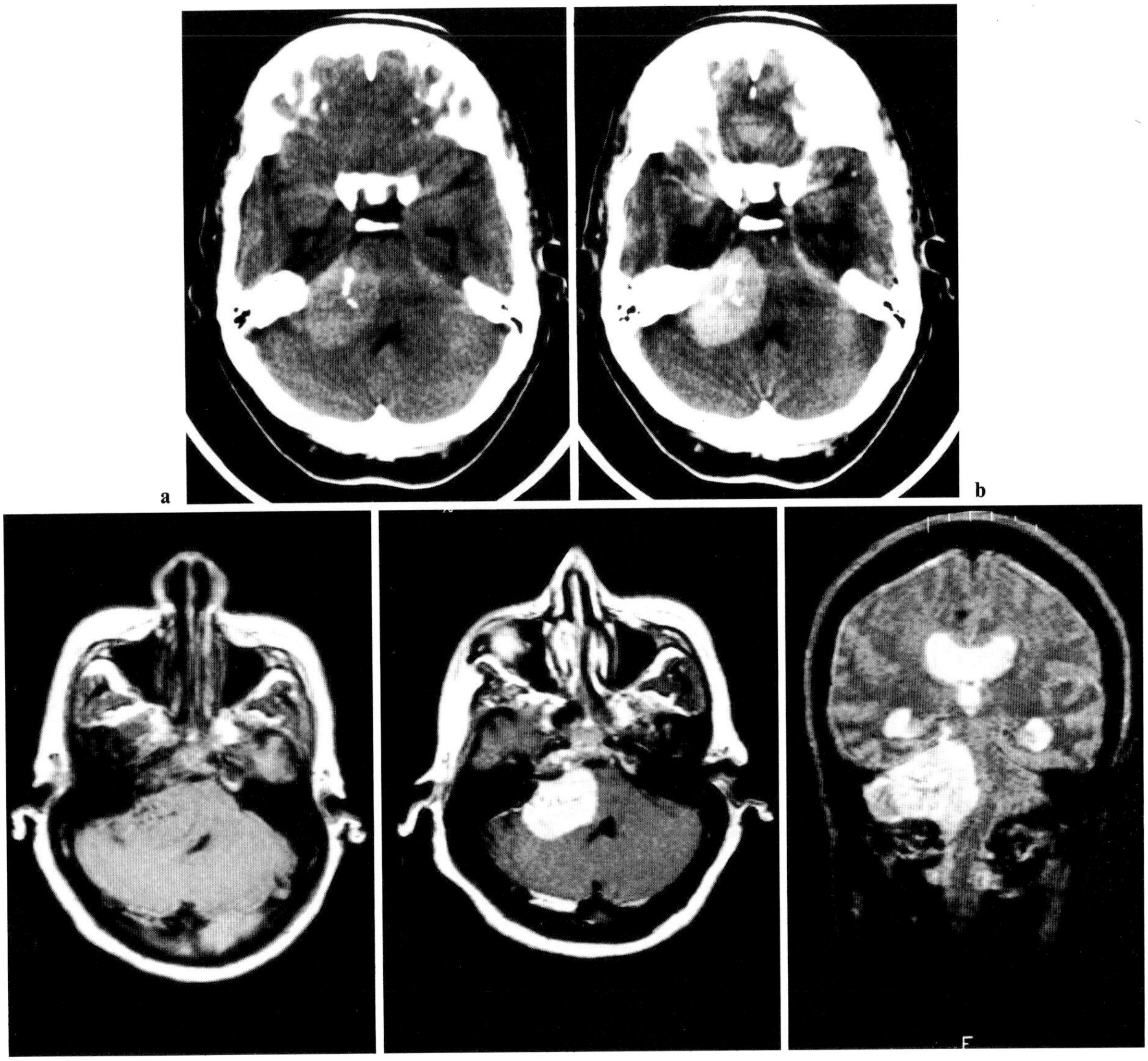

Fig. 1.8 a–e. Typical appearance of a cerebellopontine angle meningioma in nonenhanced (a), enhanced (b) axial CT scans and in axial T1-weighted (c), axial gadolinium-enhanced (d) MRI scans. A coronal T2-weighted MRI scan is also shown (e)

This same feature of MRI (poor bone imaging) may help in demonstrating small tumors in areas in which CT is prone to yield bony artifacts, such as the cerebellopontine angle [16]. Once the diagnosis is established, coronal, sagittal, and three-dimensional images using either CT or MRI are useful to help the surgeon conceptualize the three-dimensional extension and configuration of the tumor as well as (especially with MRI) in assessing the relationship between the tumor and major blood vessels [5] (Fig. 1.9).

Angiography, while no longer used as a primary diagnostic tool, retains its place as a major surgical adjuvant, showing the main tumor feeders, the patency of the major cerebral arteries, and dural sinuses (Figs. 1.10, 1.11). While dynamic MRI [3, 8] and, to a minor degree, CT scans may also show the patency of arteries and veins, we still prefer to use cerebral angiography for this because it provides an overall assessment of the intracranial circulation. In fact, selective cerebral angiography with temporary arterial occlusion using an intravascular balloon coupled with xenon CT cerebral blood flow measurements [23] helps in determining the possi-

1.9 a 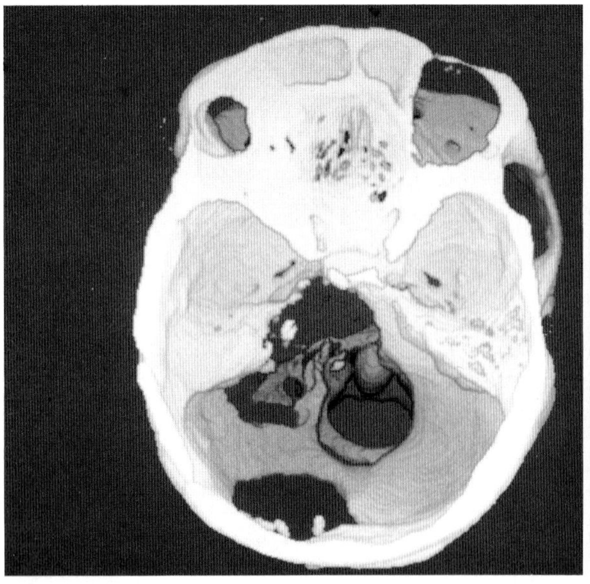 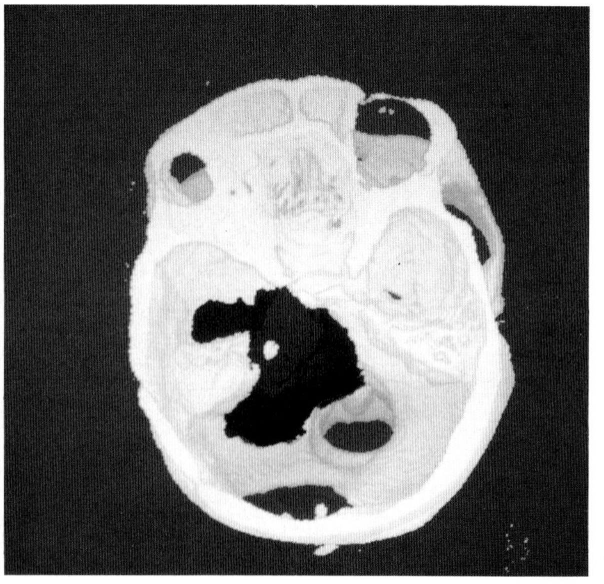 b

1.10 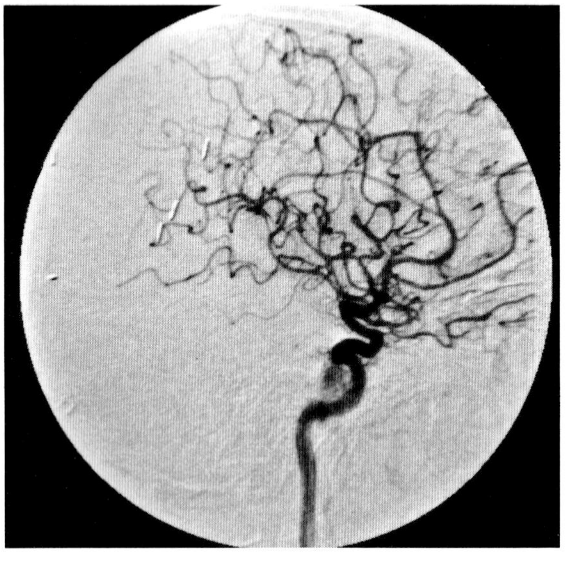

Fig. 1.9 a, b. Three-dimensional CT reconstruction of a patient with malignant meningioma with multiple intracranial locations and bony metastasis. The erosion of the clivus, petrous apex, and basiocciput is clearly evident. The bony defect in the vertical portion of the occipital squama is due to previous surgery for a suboccipital location of this malignant meningioma

Fig. 1.10. Left internal carotid artery lateral angiogram shows vascularization of clival meningioma by the meningohypophyseal artery complex

Fig. 1.11 a–g. Heavily calcified, en plaque meningioma involving the tentorium and the left cavernous sinus is shown in these CT and MRI scans. (**a** Enhanced axial CT scan. **b** T2-weighted axial MRI scan. **c** Gadolinium-enhanced sagittal MRI scan). Angiogram shows partial occlusion of the torcular, complete occlusion of the right transverse sinus, with the exception of the most proximal portion, complete occlusion of the left transverse sinus. Venous engorgement is demonstrated in the cerebellum. (**d** Right vertebral angiography, AP projection). Reverse of flow in the superior sagittal sinus that fills posterior and anteriorly emptying into a dilated left intraorbital vein is demonstrated. (**e, f** Right internal carotid angiogram, lateral view. **g** Right internal carotid angiogram, AP view)

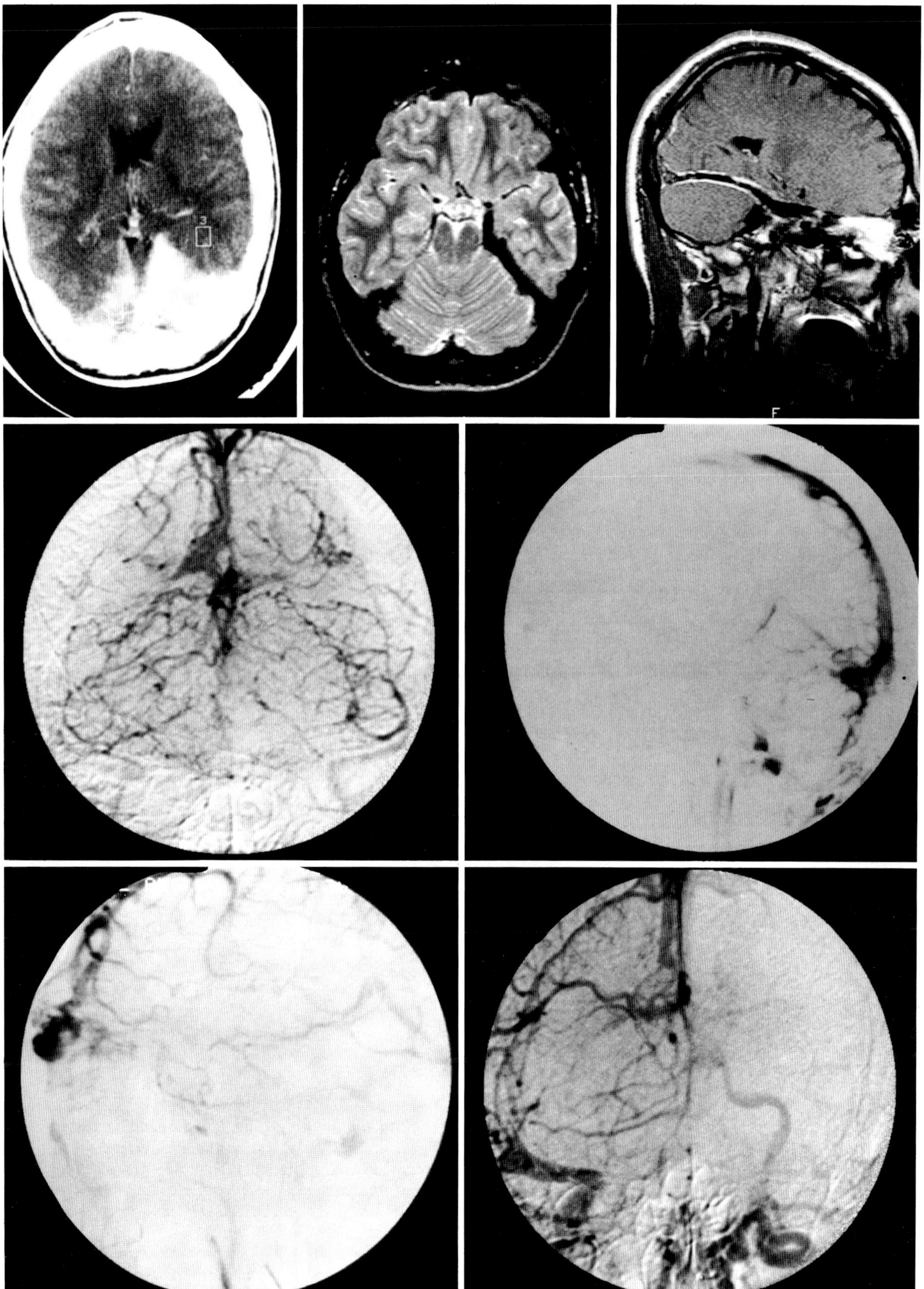

a, b c d e f g

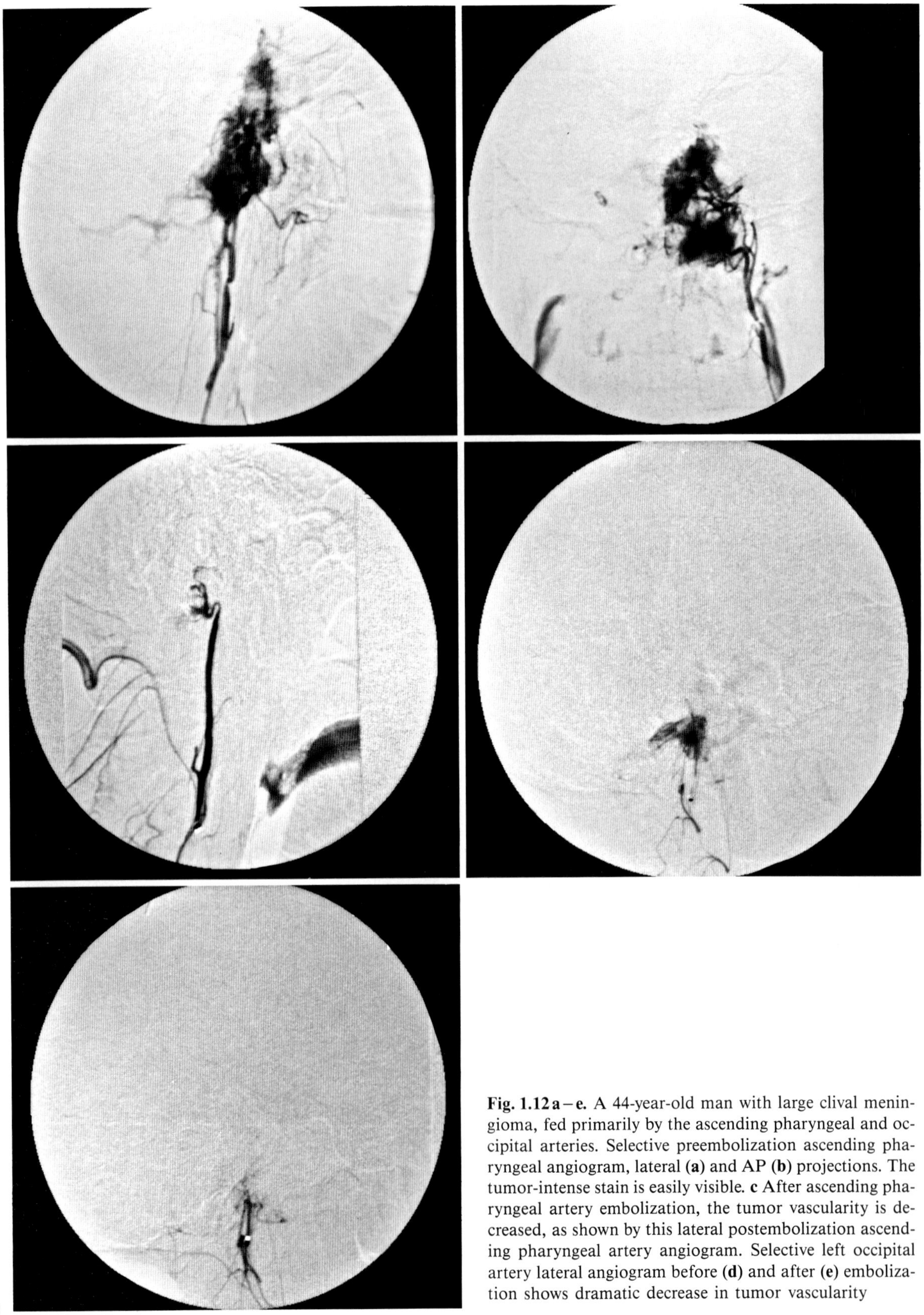

Fig. 1.12 a – e. A 44-year-old man with large clival meningioma, fed primarily by the ascending pharyngeal and occipital arteries. Selective preembolization ascending pharyngeal angiogram, lateral (**a**) and AP (**b**) projections. The tumor-intense stain is easily visible. **c** After ascending pharyngeal artery embolization, the tumor vascularity is decreased, as shown by this lateral postembolization ascending pharyngeal artery angiogram. Selective left occipital artery lateral angiogram before (**d**) and after (**e**) embolization shows dramatic decrease in tumor vascularity

ble anatomical and functional compensations of the circle of Willis when one of its major components is temporarily or permanently occluded. This information helps in better defining the goals of surgery and in selecting those patients who are candidates for a neurovascular augmentative procedure. In addition, preoperative angiography may be useful in considering, planning, and executing preoperative embolization of the lesion [19] (Fig. 1.12). However, we have not often used this preoperative embolization.

Meningiomas are usually benign tumors, and if they can be totally removed, the recurrence rate is low and the patient is often cured [24, 26]. Surgery of meningiomas in general and of skull base meningiomas in particular is difficult, and clinical judgement must be exercised in recommending surgery and, during the operation, in deciding when total removal is feasible, and if feasible, when it is advisable. Especially today, as increasing neurosurgical sophistication makes no intracranial region inaccessible – with the possibilities of cavernous sinus surgery, intrapetrous surgery, resection of intracavernous carotid artery, and petrosupraclinoid bypass, resection of cranial nerves, and nerve grafting [7, 21, 23] – it is even more important to be able to use these options with judgement and not be overwhelmed by them. The feasibility of an operation is no justification for its nonchalant performance; this is even more true with meningiomas that are generally benign lesions, whose growth potential in the individual tumor is unknown, but whose growth is generally slow. For this reason, it is sometimes preferable to remove partially even a completely resectable tumor rather than to expose the patient to an unreasonable risk. Moreover, in making a surgical decision it is important to consider that meningiomas are, at least sometimes, sensitive to conventional radiation therapy and probably even more sensitive to the newest radiation therapy delivery systems due to the increasing amount of radiation that may be concentrated on a small target [4, 23, 26].

The following chapters report our experience over the 11-year period from January 1978 to December 1988 at the Nordstadt Hospital in Hannover, Federal Republic of Germany. During this time we have treated a total of 420 patients for meningioma; 217 of these tumors were of the skull base. Table 1.1 summarizes our material in terms of tumor localization.

Table 1.1. Meningiomas: January 1978 – December 1988, Nordstadt Krankenhaus, Hannover, FRG

Skull base	217
Olfactory groove	14
Suprasellar	31
Medial sphenoid wing	27
Middle sphenoid wing	18
Lateral sphenoid wing	8
Jugular foramen	3
Low clivus + foramen magnum (craniospinal)	9
Upper + middle clivus	2
Posterior pyramid (anterior to internal auditory meatus)	32
Posterior pyramid (posterior to internal auditory meatus)	24
Petroclival	27
Incisural	4
Trigeminal	4
Cavernous sinus	1
Miscellaneous locations	9
Intraosseous	4
Intracranial, other than skull base	166
Intraorbital + optic sheath	9
Cerebral convexity	81
Parasagittal	32
Falx	27
Cerebellar convexity	11
Intraventricular	2
Pineal region	4
Spinal	37
Total	420

References

1. Bailey P, Cushing H, Eisenhardt L (1928) Angioblastic meningiomas. Arch Pathol 6:953–990
2. Borovich B, Doron Y (1986) Recurrence of intracranial meningiomas: the role played by regional multicentricity. J Neurosurg 64:58–63
3. Bradley WG (1987) Magnetic resonance appearance of flowing blood and cerebrospinal fluid. In: Brant-Zawadzki M, Norman D (eds) Magnetic resonance imaging of the central nervous system. Raven, New York, pp 83–96
4. Carella RJ, Ransohoff J, Newall J (1982) Role of radiation therapy in the management of meningiomas. Neurosurgery 10:332–339
5. Chalif DJ, Dufresne CR, Ransohoff J, McCarthy JA (1988) Three dimensional computed tomographic reconstructions of intracranial meningiomas. Neurosurgery 23:570–575

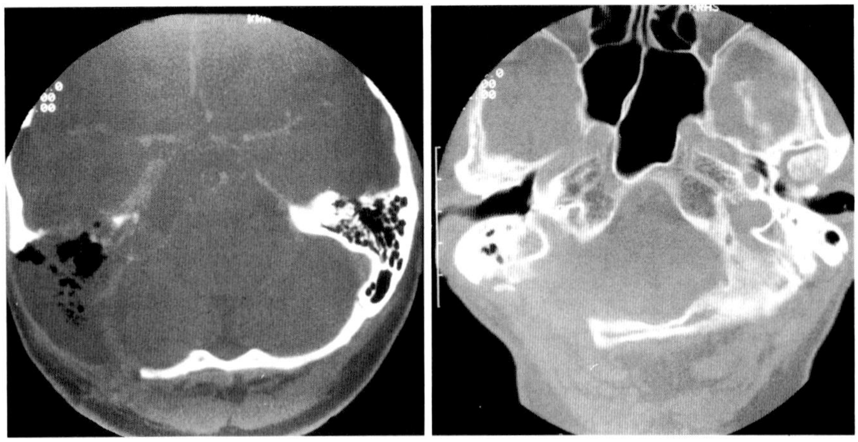

a b

Fig. 2.1 a, b. The distance from the edge of the craniectomy to the clivus is significantly less in the presigmoid sinus avenue (**a**) than in the conventional suboccipital approach (**b**)

mas, namely intratumoral (intracapsular) decompression (debulking) alternated with careful separation of the tumor from the brain and from the other vascular and neural structures that lie in the subarachnoid space, trying to develop an extraarachnoidal plane of cleavage. The dissection must proceed not only toward the brain but also toward the skull base, eventually leading to the control of the vascular pedicle of the tumor. This intratumoral debulking may be accomplished, depending on the surgeon's preference, using microsurgical instruments, ultrasound surgical aspiration, CO_2 laser, or a combination of them. While the Nd-Yag laser has been shown to be useful in the surgery of large anterior fossa basal meningiomas, its use in the posterior fossa has been associated with multiple complications as a result of brainstem injury due to the unpredictable scattering of this type of wavelength [5]. The development of the extraarachnoidal plane is better performed using microsurgical instruments, alternating microscissors with microsurgical forceps that are used to grasp and peel away the arachnoid, or, in case the arachnoid is breeched, the structures contained in the subarachnoid space. Figure 2.2 shows the instruments that we have found to be most valuable in the removal of skull base meningiomas. There is no problem in transecting, after careful coagulation, the parasitized pial vessels. Invasion of arteri-

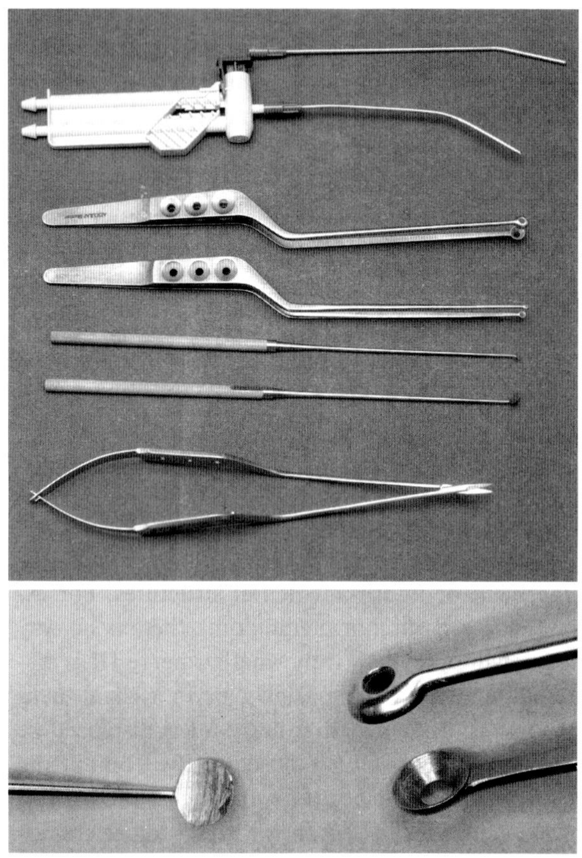

a b

Fig. 2.2 a, b. Some of the surgical instruments found particularly useful in the removal of skull base meningiomas. **a** *From top to bottom*, hydroflow suction irrigation system (Portex, Kent, UK), tumor tissue fixation forceps, round cutting knives, and dissecting scissors (Aesculap, Tuttlingen, FRG). **b** Close-up view of the basket-shaped working end of the tumor forceps and the 45° angle tumor knive

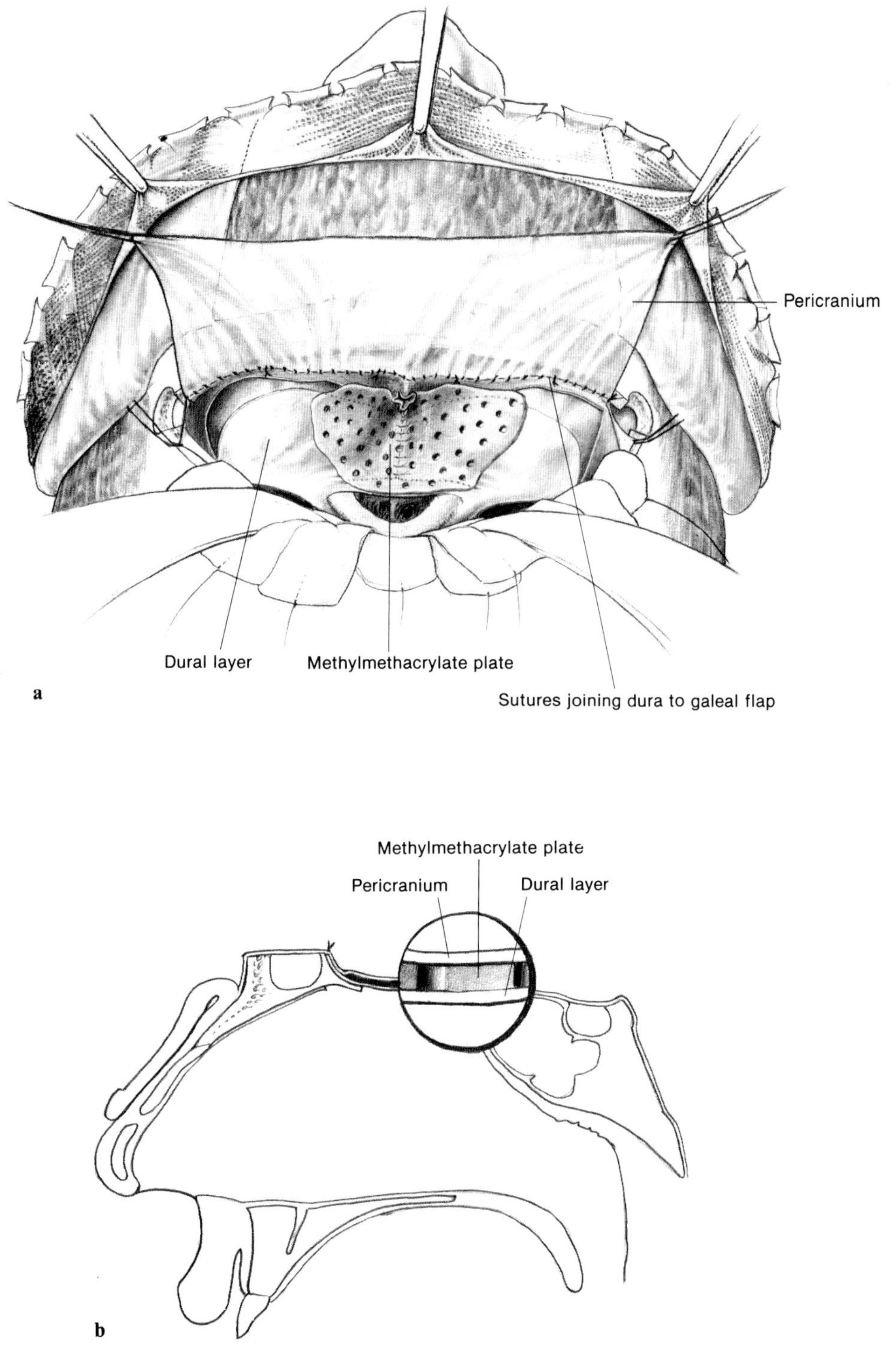

Fig. 2.3 a, b. Three-layer reconstruction of the skull base. **a** If possible, the dura of the anterior skull base is used to make rotation flaps that form the caudal layer of the reconstruction. This layer is covered by a suitably molded methylmethacrylate implant that overlaps the osseous defect. The implant is perforated for scar tissue ingrowth. The innermost layer is formed by swinging an inferiorly based galeal pericranial flap over the plastic implant. The flap is first sutured to the inferior dural margin and then fixed to the minor sphenoid wings with fibrin adhesive and posterior fixation sutures. **b** Sagittal section of the three-layer cranioplasty showing the relative positions of the dural layer, plastic implant, and galeal pericranial flap. This technique surrounds the plastic implant with viable tissue on all sides

al wall and nerves by meningiomas may occur [6]; this must be recognized intraoperatively and differentiated from the more frequent encasement of these structures by the tumor lobule and dealt with appropriately. While a structure encased by the tumor may be completely freed from it, a structure that is invaded cannot be freed from the tumor. Radicality in these cases may be achieved only by excision of the involved segment and continuity restored anatomically by the appropriate neural or vascular graft. Whether this is indicated is a matter of surgical judgement and is often a crucial intraoperative decision.

Surgery of skull base meningiomas must be considered suboptimal if the dural and bony attachment of the tumor is not dealt with effectively. In fact, it has been shown that lack of treatment of this dural matrix is associated with a recurrence rate of 30%, simple coagulation with 20%, and excision of the dura with a 10% recurrence rate [11]. It has been our observation that this dural invasion area is usually limited, even in large tumors. Wide removal of the dura must be accompanied by removal at surgery of any part of the bony skull base that is preoperatively known to be invaded by tumor, or that is even slightly suspicious, usually being irregular or hyperostotic. We recommend, whenever feasible, removal of abnormal bone and dura with some degree of margins since it has been shown that apparently normal dura surrounding the attachment of the meningioma may indeed contain meningotheliomatous cell aggregates that could perhaps represent the source of a recurrence in presumably completely resected tumors [2]. If extensive bony removal is necessary, and a paranasal sinus is entered, the skull base must be reconstructed; in its most extensive form, when paranasal sinuses are widely entered, this rebuilding of the skull base may require dural rotational flaps, acrylic, and a galea-periosteal flap [10] (Fig. 2.3). Opened mastoid cells are sealed using muscle and fibrin glue or bone wax. Dura is always closed in a water-tight fashion using, if necessary, dural substitute. Fibrin glue may be used to reinforce the dural closure. Extensive epidural dead space, such as that resulting from removal of large foramen jugulare meningioma, is obliterated using free or pedicled muscle flaps.

While meningiomas are usually globular or lobulated tumors, at times they grow diffusely in the subdural space (en plaque meningiomas) and enter all the skull base vascular and neural foramina with diffuse involvement of the dura and bone and extradural extensions, which makes their total surgical removal problematic. In our experience this type of growth has been the major obstacle to safe total surgical removal of the tumor.

References

1. Ammirati M, Samii M, Sepehrnia A (1990) Surgery of large retrochiasmatic craniopharyngiomas in children. Childs Nerv Syst 6:13–17
2. Borovich B, Doron Y (1986) Recurrence of intracranial meningiomas: the role played by regional multicentricity. J Neurosurg 64:58–63
3. Challa VR, Markesbery WR (1985) Meningiomas: pathology. In: Wilkins RH, Rengachary SS (eds) Neurosurgery. McGraw-Hill, New York, pp 613–622
4. Williams PL, Warwick R (1980) Gray's anatomy, 36th edn. Saunders, Philadelphia, p 1052
5. Jain KK (1985) Complications of use of the neodymium: yttrium aluminum garnet laser. Neurosurgery 16:759–762
6. Kepes JJ (1987) Meningiomas biology, pathology and differential diagnosis. Masseon New York, p 112
7. Moody DM (1985) Meningiomas radiology. In: Wilkins RH, Rengachary SS (eds) Neurosurgery. McGraw-Hill, New York, pp 623–634
8. Rubinstein LS (1972) Tumors of the central nervous system. AFIP, Washington, pp 169–190
9. Samii M, Ammirati M (1988) The combined supra-infratentorial presigmoid sinus avenue to the petroclival region. Surgical techniques and clinical applications. Acta Neurochir (Wien) 95:6–12
10. Samii M, Draf W (1989) Surgery of the skull base. Springer, Berlin Heidelberg New York, pp 171–177
11. Simpson D (1957) The recurrence of intracranial meningiomas after surgical treatment. J Neurol Neurosurg Psychiatry 20:22–39
12. Tenner MA (1971) The role of conventional neuroradiologic techniques in relation to computed tomography. In: Sher JH, Ford DH (eds) Primary intracranial neoplasms. Medicine and Science, New York, pp 71–85
13. Yasargil MG (1984) Microneurosurgery. Thieme, Stuttgart, p 24

CHAPTER 3

Olfactory Groove Meningiomas

General Considerations

Olfactory groove meningiomas originate from the crista galli and adjacent lamina cribrosa near the junction between the cribriform plate and the planum sphenoidale [3]. In terms of clinical presentation and size of the tumor at the time of diagnosis little can be added to Cushing's description. These tumors are still usually diagnosed when they are of a significant size, and the most common presenting symptoms are altered mental status followed by decreased vision [14]. Although anosmia and Foster-Kennedy syndrome (primary optic atrophy on the side of the lesion and contralateral papilledema) [10] are often mentioned as typical symptoms of olfactory groove meningiomas [1, 11], they are only rarely observed [6]. Anosmia was probably the presenting complaint in only three of the 29 patients reported by Cushing [3] and in none of Bakay's patients [2]. Foster-Kennedy syndrome was seen in only seven of Cushing's patients [3], and this is not surprising considering that olfactory groove meningiomas are usually bilateral. In our series anosmia was present in three patients and Foster-Kennedy syndrome in none (see "Personal Series"). As with meningiomas in any other location, olfactory groove meningiomas may attain a very large size although the patient remains asymptomatic. Cushing reported an autoptic finding in a 71-year-old man, in perfect health, with a 102-g olfactory groove meningioma, who died of kidney failure and had no neurological disturbances [3].

Olfactory groove meningiomas are of special interest to neurosurgery, first, because improvements in their surgical outcome have paralleled advances in neurosurgery (as demonstrated by the decrease in surgical mortality rate from the over 30% of Cushing [3] and others [4, 8] to the 0% of Ojemann [13] and our own series), and, second, because one of the first successful operations of an intracranial neoplasm was for an olfactory groove meningioma. In 1885 Francesco Durante, professor of clinical surgery at the University of Rome, removed, via left osteoplastic frontal craniotomy, a unilateral left 70-g olfactory groove meningioma that had caused anosmia, personality changes, and exophthalmos of more than 1-year duration in a 35-year-old woman. The operation lasted 1 h, and the patient was well at the follow-up 19 years later [5, 7].

The typical CT appearance of an olfactory groove meningioma is of an enhancing, round, anterior frontal mass, usually extending to both sides of the midline (Fig. 3.1). Enhanced MRI displays a similar picture (Fig. 3.2). An angiogram shows the typical feature of a midline subfrontal mass: elevation and stretching of the A2 segment of the anterior cerebral artery and its branches that describe a

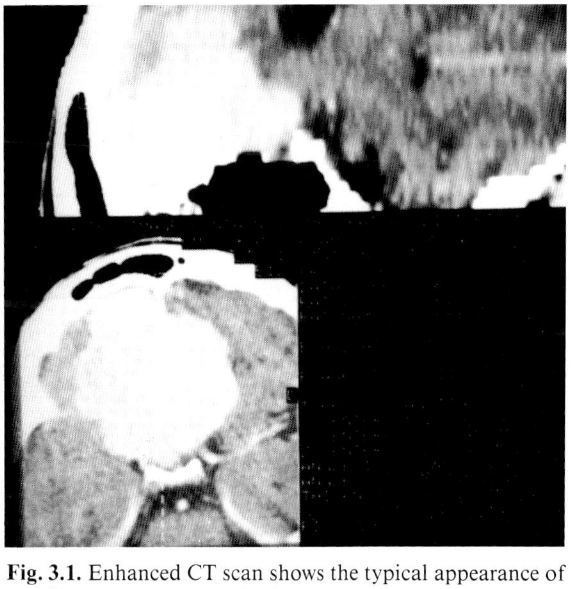

Fig. 3.1. Enhanced CT scan shows the typical appearance of an olfactory groove meningioma

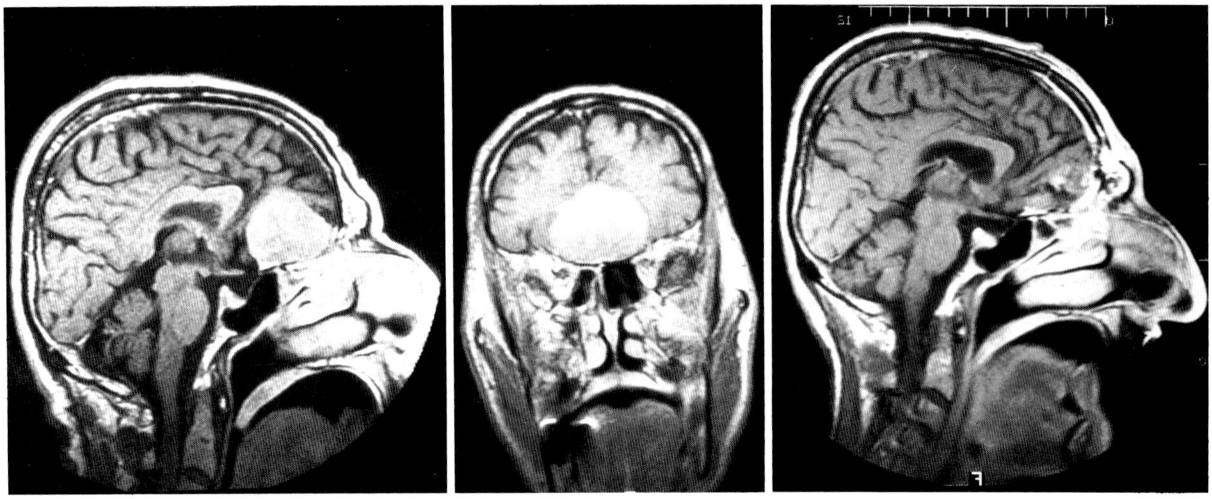

a, b c

Fig. 3.2 a–c. A 64-old man with 1-year history of progressive dementia and large olfactory groove meningioma. Gadolinium-enhanced sagittal (**a**) and coronal (**b**) MRI scans show 4×4 cm olfactory groove meningioma. **c** Postoperative sagittal gadolinium-enhanced MRI scan shows total tumor removal. The patient made an uneventful postoperative recovery

Table 3.1. Olfactory groove meningiomas

Number	14
Age: range/mean/median (years)	38 – 77/58/57
Women/men	12/2
Symptom (most common)	Personality change
Sign (most common)	Bilateral frontal lobe signs
Tumor removal	
Total	14
Subtotal	0
Outcome	
Good	11
Fair	3
Poor	0
Deaths	0

concave arc forward and downward (see Fig. 3.10c). There may also be closing of the siphon due to downward displacement of the intraarachnoidal internal carotid artery. A vascular stain may be evident as well as tumor feeders usually coming from the ophthalmic artery via ethmoidal branches.

Personal Series

Table 3.1 details our material. In this and following tables a good outcome is scored when the patient is independent, a fair outcome when he needs occasional assistance, and a poor outcome when the patient needs continuous assistance. The extent of surgical removal was assessed intraoperatively and/or postoperative enhanced CT scans. Personality change characteristic of a bifrontal lesion was the most common presenting symptom (ten patients); we observed generalized tonic clonic seizures in three. Only one patient complained of anosmia; this was detected clinically in three patients, always bilaterally. Three patients had decreased vision; none had Foster-Kennedy syndrome. In one patient the tumor extended, via the anterior fossa floor, into the sphenoid and ethmoid cavities. This tumor was removed from above, and the skull base reconstructed using a galea-periosteal flap reinforced by a lyodura layer. The three fair results were due to persistent frontal lobe signs.

Surgical Considerations

Olfactory groove meningiomas grow superiorly and posteriorly, elevating the basal frontal lobe and the A2 segments of the anterior cerebral artery. Their midline posterior extension may grow under and between the A1 segment, pushing them laterally and/or enveloping them as well as the anterior

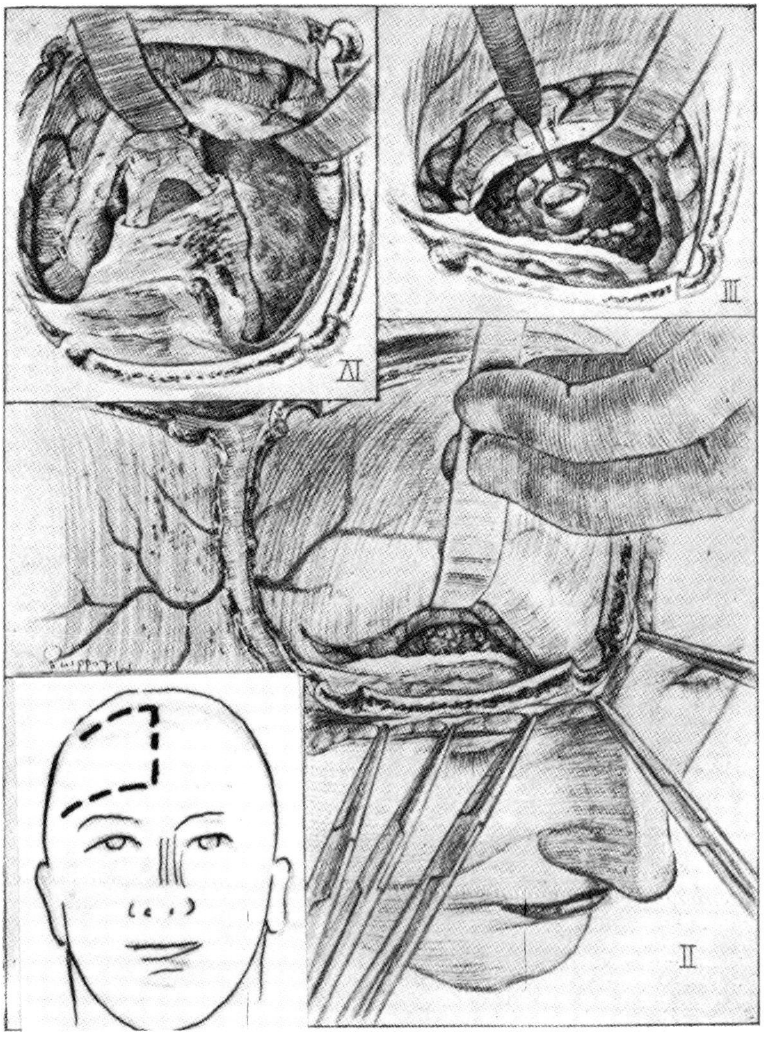

Fig. 3.3. Cushing's approach to olfactory groove meningiomas (modified from [3])

communicating artery. The optic chiasm and the optic nerves are usually depressed by olfactory groove meningiomas. Cushing approached these tumors through a right frontal osteoplastic craniotomy, with incision of the dura along the sphenoid ridge, retraction of the basal frontal lobe, removal of that part of the frontal lobe overlying the tumor, and removal of the homolateral tumor along the floor of the frontal fossa in an anteroposterior plane; providing access to the contralateral tumor was obtained after removal of the anterior portion of the falx just below the superior sagittal sinus [3] (Fig. 3.3). Kempe recommended a unilateral low frontal craniotomy on the side of the major tumor extension extending anteriorly to the midline and posteriorly to the pterion [9] (Fig. 3.4a). In the case of large tumors when a prefrontal lobectomy is planned, the frontal craniotomy is extended superiorly to incorporate the coronal suture [9] (Fig. 3.4b). The tumor is then removed, working on the lateral side of the frontal fossa in a posteroanterior direction, and the contralateral tumor is reached after removal of the falx in a way similar to that described by Cushing [3] (Fig. 3.4c). Morley recommends a bifrontal craniotomy [12], as does Ojemann [13]. MacCarty uses a unilateral frontal craniotomy for small tumors and a bifrontal craniotomy for the usual larger tumors [11].

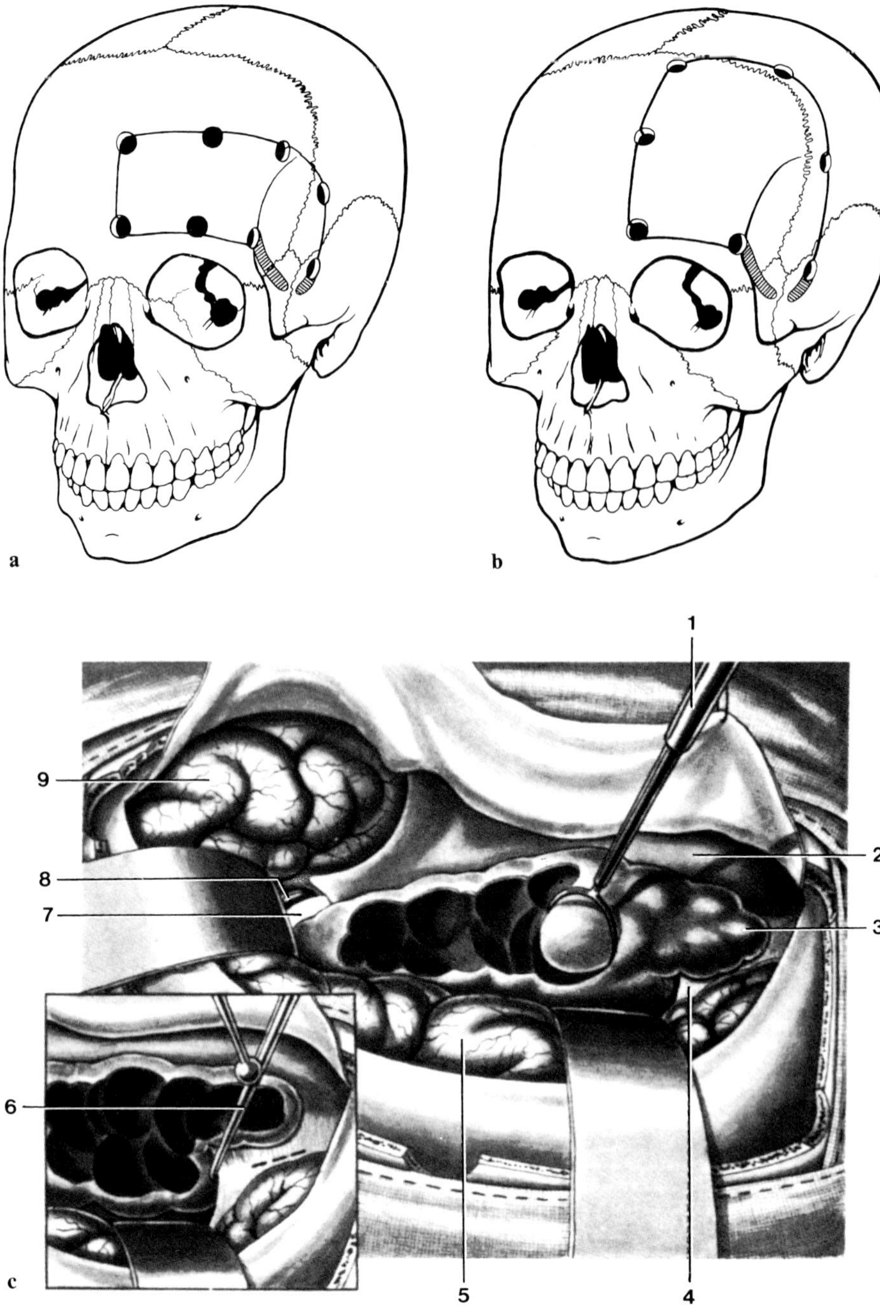

Fig. 3.4 a – c. Kempe's approach to olfactory groove meningiomas. **a** Craniotomy for smaller tumor. **b** Craniotomy for larger tumor. The skin incision is, in both instances, bicoronal. **c** Intraoperative sketch showing removal of the tumor using loop electrode. *Inset* shows removal of contralateral tumor after division of the falx cerebri. *1*, Loop electrode; *2*, frontal fossa; *3*, tumor; *4*, falx; *5*, frontal lobe; *6*, sectioning of falx; *7*, optic nerve; *8*, internal carotid artery; *9*, temporal lobe. (Modified from [9])

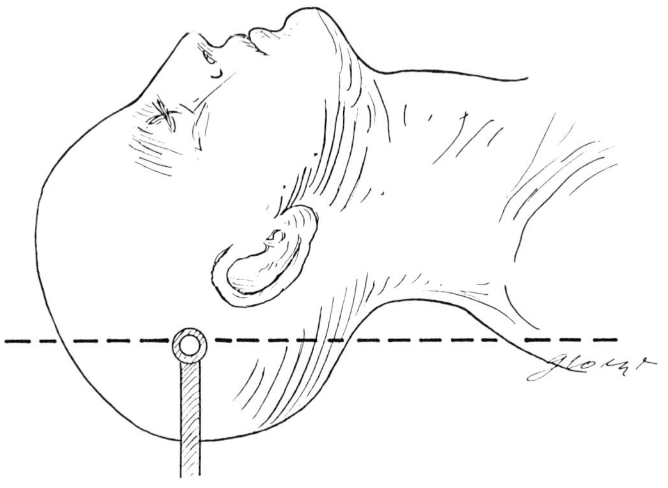

Fig. 3.5. Patient's position. Courtesy of Gwynne Gloege, Los Angeles

Since olfactory groove meningiomas usually attain a significant size before the diagnosis is made, and since they are quite invariably bilateral, we consider the approach of choice to be a bifrontal craniotomy with elevation of both frontal lobes and removal of the tumor following sagittal/parasagittal planes along both frontal fossae. We believe that the risks of bilateral frontal lobe retraction have been somewhat overstated, especially in the case of olfactory groove meningiomas. In fact, both frontal lobes have already been elevated by the tumor, as it is shown by CT and MRI scans (Figs. 3.1, 3.2) and by intraoperative inspection. There is usually only a small amount of anteromesial frontal lobe tissue covering the tumor on both sides. In addition, appropriate and timely use of osmotic diuresis, hyperventilation, and thoughtful positioning of the patient, all work to further minimize the amount of frontal lobe retraction by decreasing the brain volume (diuresis, hypocarbnia) and by letting the frontal lobe fall off the anterior fossa [15].

Finally, placing the inferior craniotomy line just above the supraorbital ridge and just above and behind the frontozygomatic suture leads to the encircling of the floor of the anterior fossa, again helping in reducing frontal lobe retraction. It is true that executing the inferior leg of the craniotomy in such a way leads almost invariably into the frontal sinus, with its possible complications (cerebrospinal fluid rhinorrhea, infection, mucocele). However, we believe that the advantages of such a craniotomy in terms of lessening frontal lobe retraction far outweigh the possible risks, which are reduced practically to zero if a systematic approach to the opened frontal sinus is taken. In this regard we recommend removal of the bony septa, together with excision of the exposed mucosa and closing of the now single sinus cavity with a pericranial flap developed from the bicoronal scalp flap.

The technique that we use in removal of olfactory groove meningiomas is the following.

Position. The patient is positioned supine with the head secured in a three-point skeletal fixation device. The head is elevated above the right atrium using the table pitch and extended at the craniocervical junction. Extension of the head provides gravitational retraction of the frontal lobes that fall away from the anterior skull base, lessening the amount of frontal lobe retraction (Fig. 3.5).

Skin Flap. The skin incision extends from just above one zygoma to the other, approximately 1 cm in front of the tragus. At the level of the midline the incision is curved in an anteriorly convex horseshoe fashion (Fig. 3.6). Care is taken at the lateral edge of the incision to avoid injuring the superficial temporal artery or the frontotemporal branches of the facial nerve for the frontal muscle. We prefer to reflect the periosteum together with the scalp flap to be used later as a pedicled galea-periosteal flap to cover the opened frontal sinus. Subperiosteal dissection helps in avoiding injury to the branch of the facial nerve supplying the frontal muscle; this

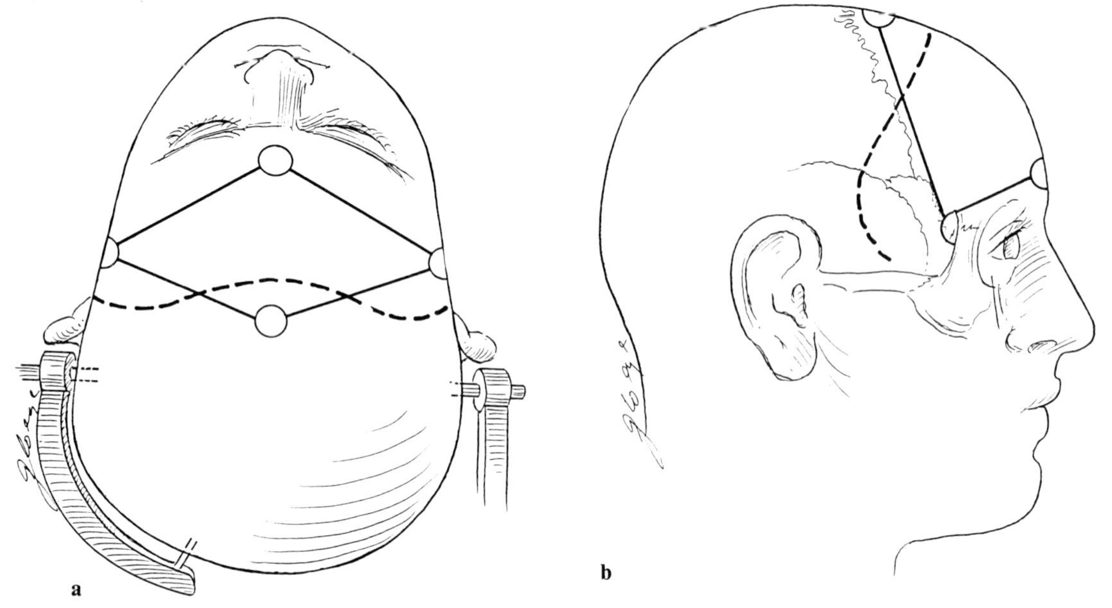

Fig. 3.6 a, b. Skin incision and craniotomy. Courtesy of Gwynne Gloege, Los Angeles

branch runs in the subcutaneous tissue underneath the galea.

The anterior portion of the temporal muscle is cut in line with the lateral portion of the scalp incision and, after separation from the anterior portion of the superior temporal line and from the posterior edge of the zygomatic process of the frontal bone, is reflected with it. Such an executed scalp flap allows for exposure of the whole anteroinferior frontal bone, including the supraorbital ridges and the glabella in the midline and the zygomatic processes laterally. Incidentally, it should be noted that when the posterior limb of the cut temporal muscle is separated from the temporal squama and retracted posteriorly, such a flap exposes the pterional region on both sides, lending itself to the execution of a bifrontopterional craniotomy.

Craniotomy. The goal of the craniotomy (Fig. 3.6) is to encircle as low as possible the entire floor of the anterior cranial fossa from one lesser sphenoid wing to the other and to elevate a flap of frontal bone to allow for retraction of both frontal lobes. This must be accomplished without placing unsightly burrholes or bone cuts across the forehead and without injuring the superior sagittal sinus. Opening of the frontal sinus is of secondary importance. All this is accomplished by placing two burrholes in the lateral frontal bone just above the frontozygomatic suture and just below the linea temporalis (keyhole). Directing these burrholes superiorly and posteriorly prevents entering of the orbit while leading exactly at or very close to the lateral extent of the ala minor. Another situation that could lead to injury of the dura or periorbita may develop when one-half of the perforator is still in bone while the other half is over the dura or the periorbita; executing the drilling in two or three states while visually checking the bony removal already accomplished each time may reduce the frequency of this complication. These lateral burrholes are then extended anteriorly for a short distance using Kerrisons. A third burrhole is placed in the midline over the superior sagittal sinus immediately behind the hairline. A fourth burrhole is placed at the glabella, and this usually enters the frontal sinus. After careful dural separation the burrholes are connected with a craniotome, trying to bevel the cut as much as possible and to connect the outer perimeters of the holes so as to have the widest possible exposure. First, the lateral burrholes are connected, with the glabellar one cutting just above the supraorbital ridge. Due to the presence of irregular bony projections in the region of the midline and to the presence of the frontal sinus it is not always possible to complete the cut with the craniotome; a high-speed drill or a bone-biting instrument may need to be used. Then the lateral burrholes are connected to the posterior midline burrhole; this must be preceded by careful dural separation from the bone in correspondence to the superior sagittal sinus and 2 cm lateral to it on each side. The bone flap is then elevated as a free flap.

Management of the Frontal Sinus. Occasionally it is possible to enter at the glabella only the anterior wall of the sinus without injuring the mucosa. In this rare situation the intact mucosa may be separated from the sinus and folded inferiorly. Usually the mucosa is injured in at least some places. It is therefore necessary to remove the exposed mucosa and to create a single bony cavity in correspondence to the exposed sinus by carefully burring away all the bony projections that usually tend to compartmentalize the sinus. When such a bony removal is conducted carefully, and when all the exposed mucosa is removed, the risks of a postoperative mucocele are significantly reduced. Later, at the end of the tumor removal, the open cavity of the sinus is closed by covering it with a pedicled galea-periosteal flap developed from the bicoronal scalp flap and sutured to the midline low basal frontal dura (Fig. 3.8).

Dural Opening. After placing tack-up sutures, the dura is cut horizontally as low as possible on each side of the midline, leaving a few millimeters of uncut dura corresponding to the superior sagittal sinus. The superior sagittal sinus is then divided between two silk sutures. The dura posterior to the superior sagittal sinus in the midline, the falx cerebri, is then cut in an anteroposterior direction under visual control, in order not to injure the anterior cerebral artery, back to its free edge. There may be some venous bleeding at this time due to the inferior sagittal sinus; this is easily controlled with bipolar coagulation. The rest of the operation up to the end of tumor removal is performed with the help of the operating microscope. The operating microscope used in all the operations described in this book was a Zeiss Contravas OPMI 6 ceiling-mounted operating microscope with a 250-mm objective lens (Carl Zeiss, Oberkochen, FRG).

Tumor Removal. After insertion of the self-retaining retractors the frontal lobes are retracted laterally and posteriorly, exposing the tumor in the midline (Fig. 3.7a). Due to the usually large size of these tumors no attempt is made at this time to dissect it away from the skull base or from the brain; rather, using bipolar coagulation, ultrasound surgical aspiration, or laser, the tumor is decompressed internally, transforming a larger tumor into a smaller one. This allows the outer part of the tumor, the tumor capsule, to fall away from the skull base and from the arachnoidal interface. As the tumor is progressively reduced in size, it can be folded and carefully separated from the skull base and brain using dissectors and cottonoids. Attempts should be made to expose and to coagulate the tumor feeders coming from the midline of the frontal fossa in the region of the lamina cribrosa. This devascularization of the tumor greatly facilitates further removal of the neoplasm. Although large meningiomas parasitize pial vessels, we think it is conceptually safer to consider all arteries stretched over the tumor as brain arteries and consequently, whenever possible, to move them away from the tumor using microforceps. As one approaches the posterior part of the tumor, the A2 segments of the anterior cerebral arteries and their branches are seen and carefully preserved. The most difficult part of the operation comes at the very end when one must deal with the posteroinferior knob of the tumor, depressing the optic nerves and chiasm and growing under and at times encircling the proximal segments of the anterior cerebral arteries and the anterior communicating artery (Fig. 3.7b). This posterior knob of the tumor, whose potential for causing trouble was recognized by Cushing [3], must be approached under direct vision; under no circumstance must this knob of tumor be delivered in the operative field by pulling on it, as the proximal anterior cerebral artery may be pulled and torn with it. The amount of frontal lobe retraction may be temporarily increased, as well as the head extension, using at the most the gravitational retraction of the frontal lobes. In such a way one may attack this portion of the tumor not only from the midline but also bilaterally after having identified the anterior clinoid processes and the proximal optic nerves. At times it may be necessary to work in the interopticocarotid space so as to dislodge knobs of

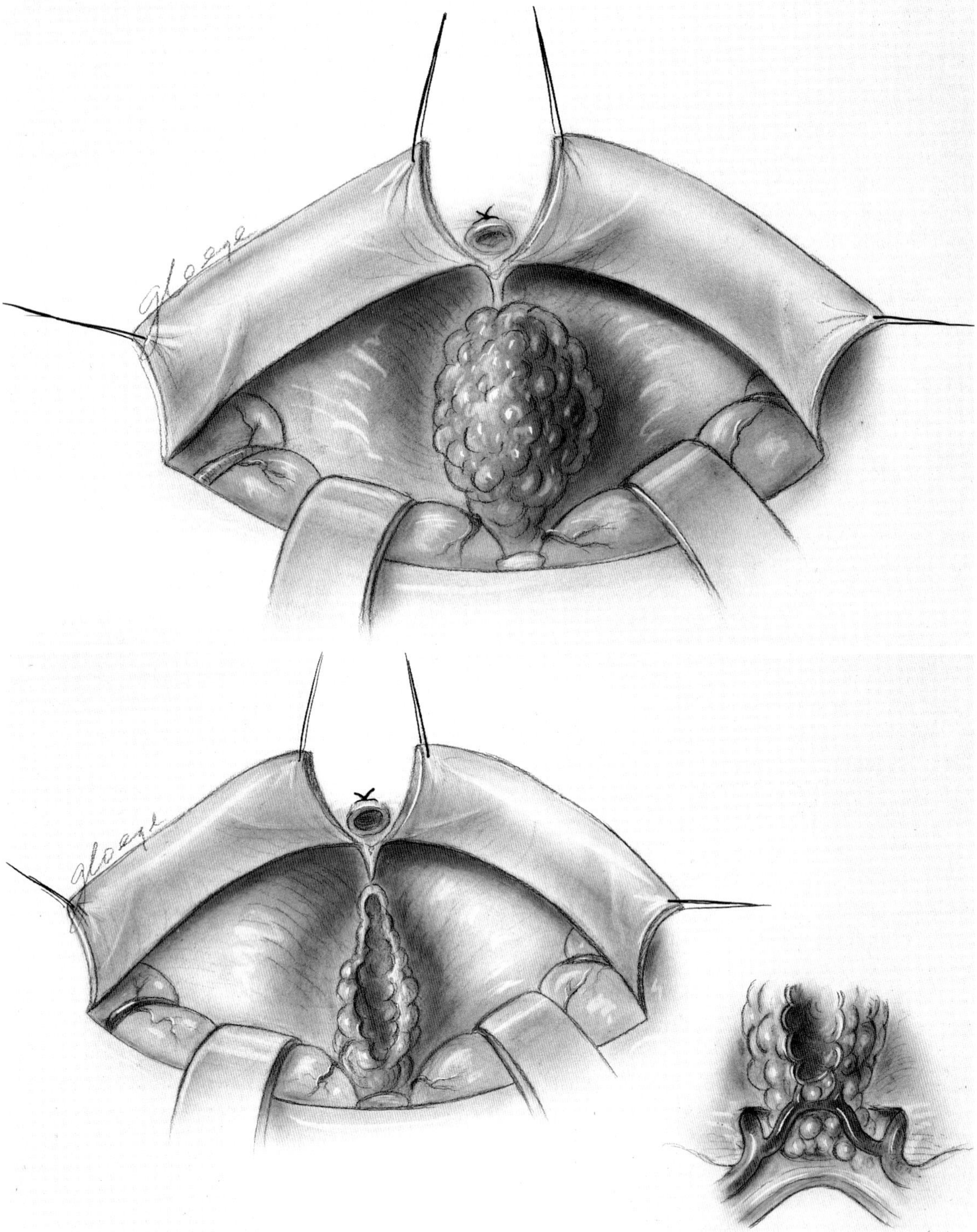

a

b

Fig. 3.7 a, b. Tumor removal. **a** The tumor is exposed in the midline after retraction of both frontal lobes. **b** The tumor is being debulked from within. *Inset* shows the close relationships between the posterior knob of the tumor and the anterior cerebral arteries complex. Courtesy of Gwynne Gloege, Los Angeles

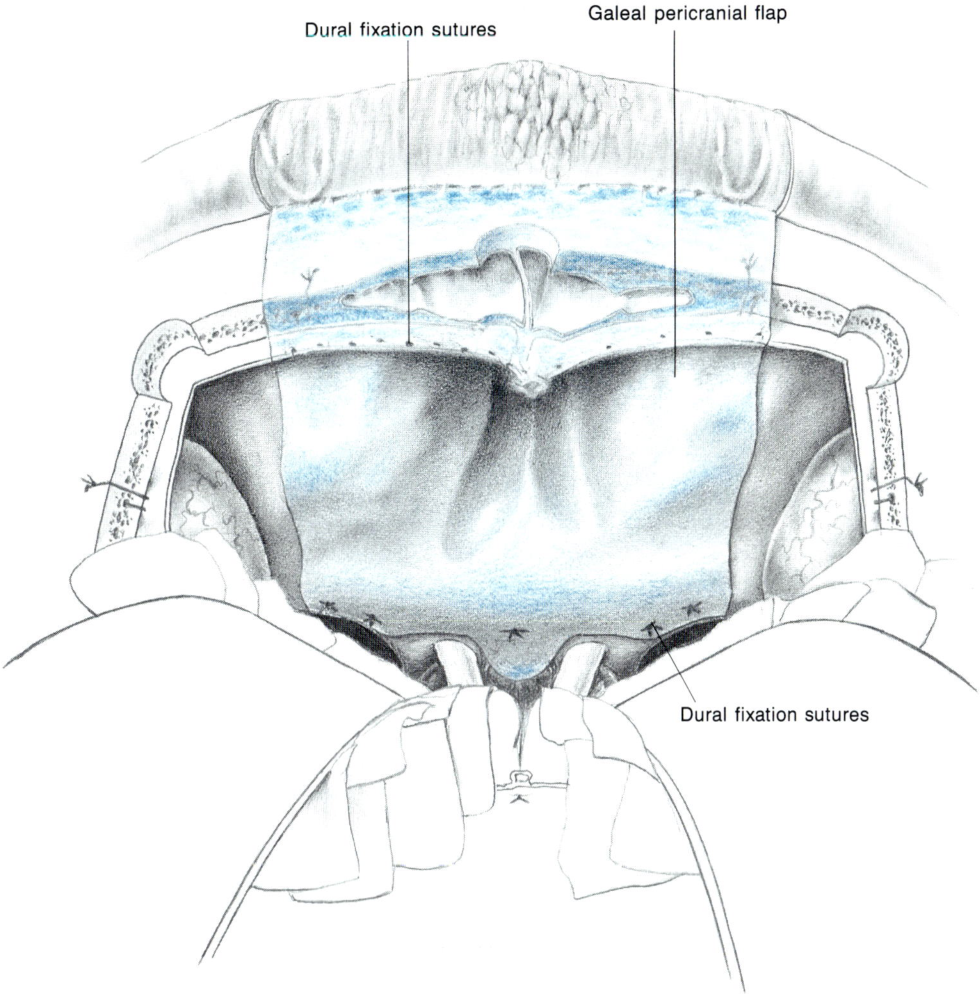

Fig. 3.8. Obliteration of the frontal sinus. An inferiorly based galeal-pericranial flap is mobilized and sutured first to the anterior cut edge of the dura, sealing off the frontal sinuses from the cranial cavity. The flap is then sutured to the posterior edge of the planum sphenoidale and lesser sphenoid wings. The flap may be additionally secured using fibrin glue. Adhesive may also be used to attach a tongue of the galeal-pericranial flap to the posterior wall of the sphenoid sinus

tumor lying lateral to the optic nerves. It is at this stage of the operation that we feel the advantages of a multiangled exposure permitted by bilateral frontal lobe retraction to be invaluable. Once the tumor has been completely removed, one excises the dural area of attachment, on the lamina cribrosa. If the bone is involved, it is removed with a high-speed drill. In the usual situation the skull base is reconstructed using a pericranial graft held in place by sutures reinforced with fibrin glue [16] (Fig. 3.8). If the amount of bony removal is greater than usual, and if the paranasal cavities are entered, the pericranial graft must be reinforced with a lyodura graft, and, in the case of extensive bone removal, rotational dural flaps are developed from the basal healthy dura, swung across the midline over the defect, and sutured to each other; acrylic may then be placed above this dural layer, and a galea-periosteal flap is placed over the anterior skull base covering the acrylic as well as the denuded area of bone from which the rotational dural flaps have been developed. If desired, a pedicled myofascial flap developed from the temporal muscle may also be used to further reinforce the reconstruction [16] (Fig. 3.9). However, each situation must be assessed individually; whatever reconstruc-

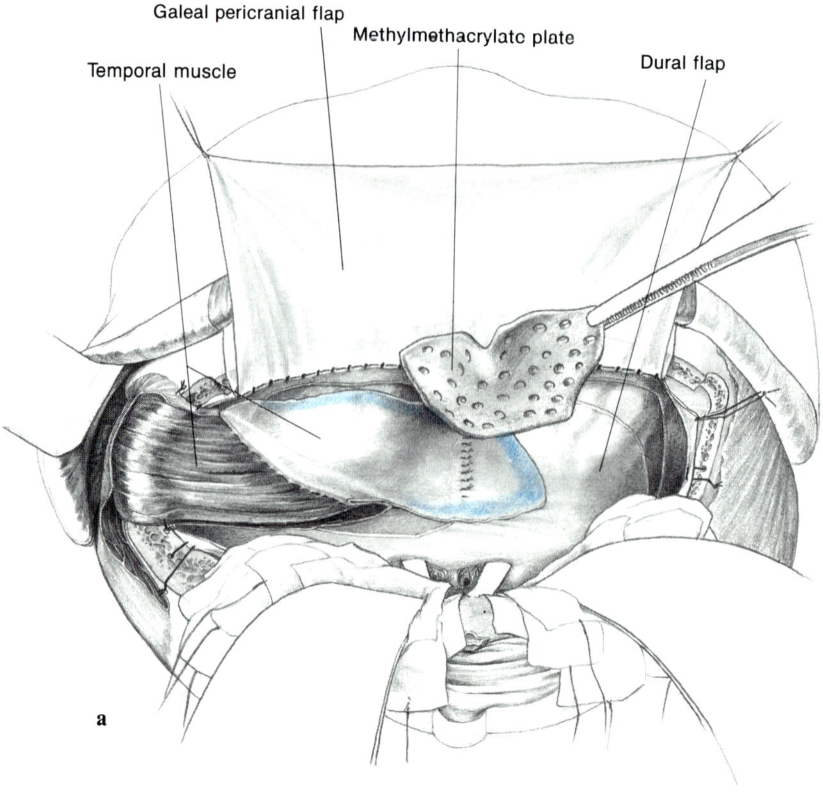

a

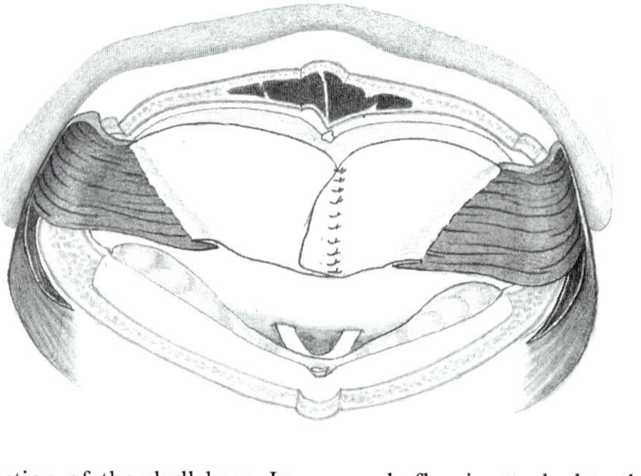

b

Fig. 3.9 a, b. Extensive reconstruction of the skull base. In extreme cases, where it is necessary to extensively resect the skull base and the dura, the caudal layer of the reconstruction may consist of temporal muscle. The outer aponeurotic layer is stripped upward, effectively doubling the muscle length. A portion of the temporal bone is removed, and the muscle flap is attached to the skull base with adhesive and additionally fixed with sutures. Retraction of the muscle is prevented by fixing it to the bone margins. If a galeal pericranial flap is not available for covering the plastic plate, the contralateral temporal muscle may be mobilized as a substitute

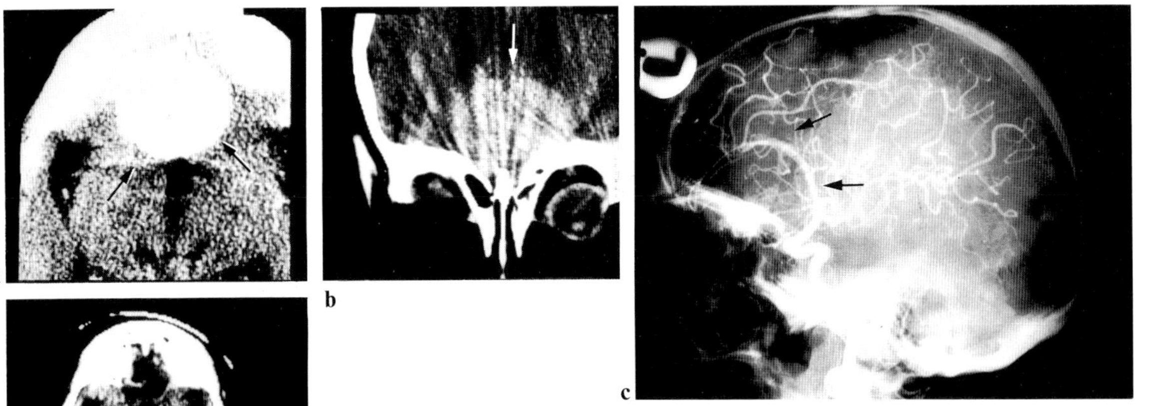
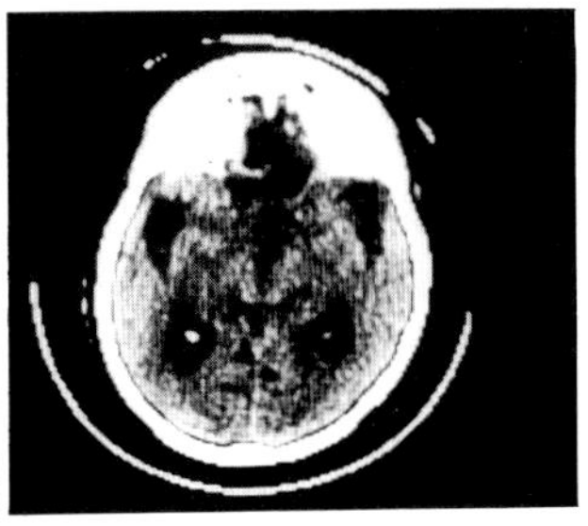

Fig. 3.10 a – d. Olfactory groove meningioma in a 59-year-old woman, preoperative and postoperative views. Preoperative axial (**a**) and coronal (**b**) CT scans demonstrate the extensive tumor (*arrows*). **c** Internal carotid angiogram shows the typical arching and posterior deviation of the anterior cerebral artery caused by the subfrontal mass. **d** Postoperative CT scan confirms the complete removal of the tumor

tion is chosen we recommend never using a nonviable material (lyodura, acrylic) immediately above a paranasal sinus and never using nonviable materials in two adjacent layers.

Illustrative Case

A 59-year-old woman presented with a 2-year history of progressive dementia. Clinical examination disclosed bilateral anosmia and a concentric contraction of the left visual field with visual acuity reduced to 20%. Plain radiographs showed erosion of the cribriform plate, and CT scans demonstrated a large mass lesion suspicious for meningioma (Fig. 3.10a, b). The angiogram showed elevation of the anterior cerebral arteries and pathological staining of the tumor vessels supplied via the ophthalmic arteries (Fig. 3.10c). The tumor was approached through a bifrontal craniotomy and exposed by gentle retraction of the frontal lobes. Piecemeal removal of the highly vascular tumor was accomplished by bipolar coagulation and resection. Both anterior cerebral arteries, the optic nerves, and the optic chiasm were microsurgically freed of tumor. After removal of the dura bordering on the tumor, the thickened crista galli and cribriform plate were removed with the diamond burr. The small skull base defect was closed in two layers with a dural graft and a galeal pericranial flap. The postoperative course was uncomplicated, and CT scans confirmed total tumor removal (Fig. 3.10d). One year later the patient was clinically asymptomatic and recurrence-free.

References

1. Adams RD, Victor M (1989) Principles of neurology, 4th edn. McGraw-Hill, New York, p 543
2. Bakay L (1984) Olfactory meningiomas. The missed diagnosis. JAMA 251:53–56
3. Cushing H, Eisenhardt C (1962) Meningiomas. Their classification, regional behavior, life history and surgical end results. Hafner, New York, pp 250–282
4. Dickel E (1957) Klinik und operative Behandlung der supratentoriellen Meningeome. Inaugural dissertation (Thesis). University of Cologne, Cologne
5. Durante F (1885) Estirpazione di un tumore endocranico (forma morbosa prima e dopo l'operazione). Boll R Acad Med (Roma) 11:247–252
6. Glaser JS (1978) Neuro-ophthalmology. Harper, Hagerstown, p 143
7. Guidetti B (1983) Francesco Durante June 29, 1844 to October 2, 1934. Surg Neurol 20:1–3
8. Holub K (1956) Intrakranielle Meningeome. Acta Neurochir (Wien) 4:355–401
9. Kempe L (1968) Operative neurosurgery, vol 1. Springer, Berlin Heidelberg New York, pp 104–108
10. Kennedy F (1911) Retrobulbar neuritis as an exact diagnostic sign of certain tumors and abscesses in the frontal lobes. Am J Med Sci 142:355–368
11. MacCarty CS, Piepgras DG, Ebersold NJ (1982) Meningeal tumors of the brain. In: Youmans J (ed) Neurologi-

cal surgery: a comprehensive reference guide to the diagnosis and management of neurosurgical problems, 2nd edn. Saunders, Philadelphia, pp 2936–2966
12. Morley TP (1973) Tumors of the cranial meninges. In: Youmans J (ed) Neurological surgery: a comprehensive reference guide to the diagnosis and management of neurosurgical problems, 1st edn. Saunders, Philadelphia, pp 1388–1411
13. Ojemann RG (1985) Clinical features and management of meningiomas. In: Wilkins RH, Rengachary SS (eds) Neurosurgery. McGraw-Hill, New York, pp 635–654
14. Ojemann RG, Swann KW (1988) Surgical management of olfactory groove, suprasellar and medial sphenoid wing meningiomas. In: Schmidek HH, Sweet WH (eds) Operative neurosurgical techniques: indications, methods and results, vol 1, 2nd edn. Grune and Stratton, New York, pp 531–545
15. Raimondi AJ (1987) Pediatric neurosurgery. Theoretic principles. Art of surgical technique. Springer, Berlin Heidelberg New York, pp 17–21
16. Samii M, Draf W (1989) Surgery of the skull base. Springer, Berlin Heidelberg New York, pp 171–177

CHAPTER 4

Suprasellar Meningiomas

General Considerations

Suprasellar meningiomas originate most frequently from the planum sphenoidale or tuberculum sellae, but they may also originate from the diaphragma sellae or anterior clinoid region. Cushing coined the term chiasmal syndrome to describe the complex of symptoms and signs commonly associated with these lesions: "primary optic atrophy with bitemporal field defects in adult patients showing an essentially normal sella turcica" [2]. Visual symptoms are still the most common presenting symptoms on admission, and the most common first symptom followed by headache [4]. Visual symptoms are asymmetric, starting in one eye, worsening in it, and spreading to the other eye, usually in the form of severe visual loss in the initial eye and decreased acuity in the opposite temporal field [3]. Signs on admission parallel the symptoms with visual signs (visual field defects, loss of visual acuity, optic atrophy) present in almost all patients [11]. In one recent series hypo-osmia was the second most common sign on admission (24%), followed by abnormal mental status and pyramidal signs, with a frequency of 9% each [12]. It is distressing that 38% of the patients were diagnosed more than 2 years after the beginning of their visual problems [14]. Due to the more immediate relationship that suprasellar meningiomas have with the optic apparatus, these tumors are diagnosed earlier, though of a relative smaller size, than olfactory groove meningiomas originating less than 2 cm anteriorly. In our series the median interval between the onset of symptoms and the diagnosis was 1 year in suprasellar meningiomas and 2 years in olfactory groove meningiomas.

The CT scan usually shows an homogeneously enhancing lesion centered on the planum sphenoidalis or on the tuberculum sellae (Fig. 4.1). In small tumors the mass may be seen originating from the anterior clinoid process and extending into the suprasellar space. Enhanced MRI scans confirm the CT findings (Fig. 4.2). Angiography shows the suprasellar mass findings: stretching and elevation of A1, closing of the siphon, and arching of A2 (Fig. 4.3).

Personal Series

Table 4.1 summarizes our clinical data. Tumor size ranged from 3 to 8 cm. Decreased vision was the most common presenting symptom and was present for a period ranging from a few weeks to 5 years (median 1 year). Three patients were blind in one eye and had severely compromised vision in the other. Postoperatively, vision was improved in 12 patients, unchanged in 8, and worse in 9. The two subtotal tumor removals were due to an en plaque type of tumor diffusely infiltrating the dura; one of these patients had already been operated on previously twice. Postoperative liquor fistula requiring reoperation was observed in three patients. One of

Table 4.1. Suprasellar meningiomas

Number	31
Age; range/mean/median (years)	5–84/52/53
Women/men	26/5
Symptom (most common)	Decreased vision
Sign (most common)	Decreased visus
Tumor removal	
Total	29
Subtotal	2
Outcome	
Good	27
Fair	2
Poor	0
Deaths	2

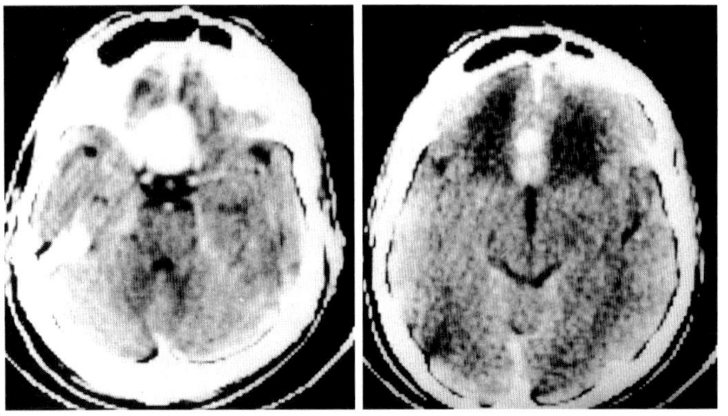

4.1 a, b

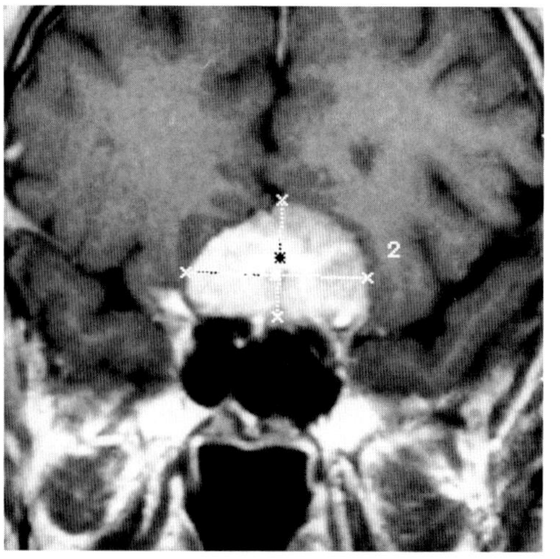

4.2

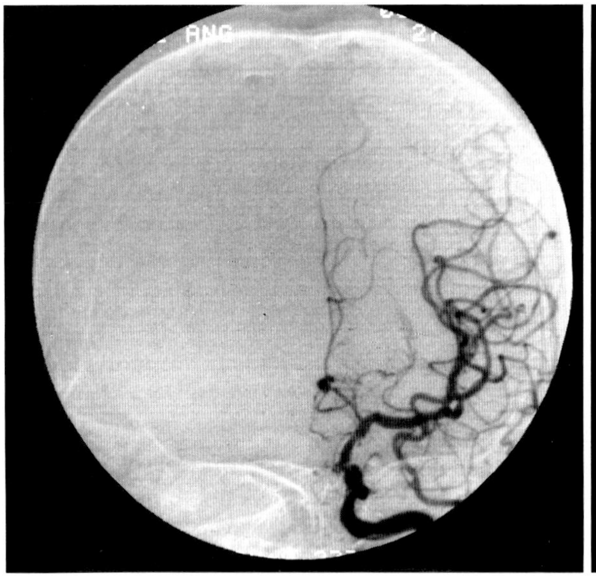

4.3 a

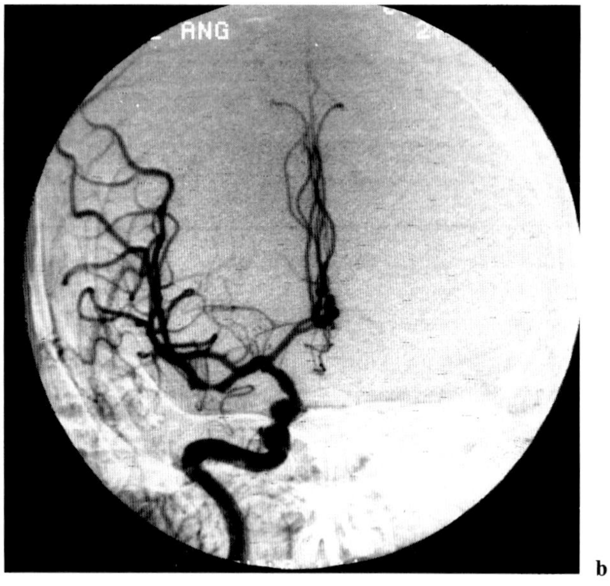

b

Fig. 4.1. **a** Enhanced CT scan of a suprasellar meningioma involving the tuberculum sellae-planum sphenoidale region and extending to the cristal galli. **b** There is marked perifocal edema

Fig. 4.2. Gadolinium-enhanced coronal MRI scan of a suprasellar meningioma

Fig. 4.3 a, b. Carotid angiograms show elevation of the A1 segment of the anterior cerebral arteries and lateral displacement and straightening of the supraclinoid internal carotid arteries. **a** AP left. **b** AP right the two deaths was due to a diencephalic insult and the other to massive postoperative edema. Of the 29 survivors 27 were fully independent.

Surgical Considerations

Suprasellar meningiomas most often originate from the planum sphenoidalis or tuberculum sellae. At least in the beginning they grow posteriorly, displacing the chiasm posteriorly and the optic nerves laterally. As their size increases they may grow in the interopticocarotid space, displacing the internal carotid artery laterally, the A1 segment upward, growing above and below the optic nerves and chiasm, and displacing or enveloping the anterior communicating artery. When they attain giant size they may "explode" from the suprasellar region, invaginating the floor of the third ventricle, eventually obstructing the foramen of Monro, and growing posteriorly pushing the pituitary stalk backward or to one side, growing into the interpeduncular region, but usually not transgressing Lillequist's membrane. Occasionally a suprasellar meningioma presents as a pure retrochiasmatic lesion [5].

Cushing approached these tumors through a right frontal craniotomy similar to the one described in Chap. 3 [2]. Kempe used a right frontotemporal craniotomy, reaching the tumor along the lesser wing of the sphenoid after retraction of the frontal and temporal lobe [7]. Ojemann recommends a frontotemporal craniotomy executed on the right side except when the tumor originates from the left anterior clinoid process; a bifrontal craniotomy is adviced for large tumors [11]. MacCarty used the frontotemporal approach, the side being determined by the major tumor bulk or by the side of greatest visual loss, with a bifrontal craniotomy being reserved only for very large tumors [9]. Morley and Kadis used a bifrontal craniotomy [6]. Logue and Symon reached the tumor going subfrontally along the midline after turning a right frontal flap and resection of the most anterior portion of the frontal lobe in large tumors [8, 13]. Al Mefty, reporting on 17 large suprasellar meningiomas, used bifrontal flap with a bilateral subfrontal approach 11 times, a right subfrontal flap 2 times, and a frontotemporal flap 4 times [1]. We believe that since these tumors are midline-suprasellar tumors, they are best and most safely approached through a bifrontal craniotomy with elevation of both frontal lobes, reaching the tumors along sagittal and parasagittal planes. This approach allows the surgeon to deal with the planum sphenoidalis portion of the tumor from the midline as well as from the right and from the left of it. More importantly, when the bulk of the tumor is removed, one may deal with the tumor involving the optic nerve, chiasm, anterior communicating artery, A1 segment, and supraclinoid internal carotid artery from different angles, namely between the optic nerves, lateral to them (interopticocarotid space), and lateral to the internal carotid artery. The bifrontal approach is recommended irrespective of the tumor size as long as it is a midline suprasellar tumor. In the rare case of a small tumor centered in the region of the anterior clinoid process we prefer a frontotemporal approach homolateral to the side of the tumor. For a description of the frontotemporal approach see Chap. 5. When using the bilateral subfrontal approach, the patient's position, scalp flap, craniotomy, brain retraction, and handling of the frontal sinus are as described in Chap. 3, the only difference being that the olfactory bulbs and tracts may be sharply separated from the olfactory sulci on the basal frontal lobes all the way back to the point at which the olfactory tract crosses the optic nerve (Fig. 4.4).

Tumor removal is performed, again, by effecting an intratumoral decompression, thus converting a large tumor into a smaller one. This tumor reduction is usually accomplished using the ultrasonic aspirator and by bipolar coagulation of small bits of tumor followed by cutting it with microscissors. In these tumors it is usually possible relatively early in the course of the procedure to reach the main feeders coming from the posterior ethmoidal area. We recommend that this be done immediately following initial intratumoral decompression, which greatly facilitates lifting of the tumor from the skull base, thus giving access to its feeders that are promptly coagulated and transsected under direct vision. This devascularization of the tumor helps in facilitating further tumor removal with acceptable blood loss (Fig. 4.5a, b). While removal of the tumor from the A2 segment is not particularly difficult, great care must be exercised in freeing the tumor from the anterior communicating artery, from

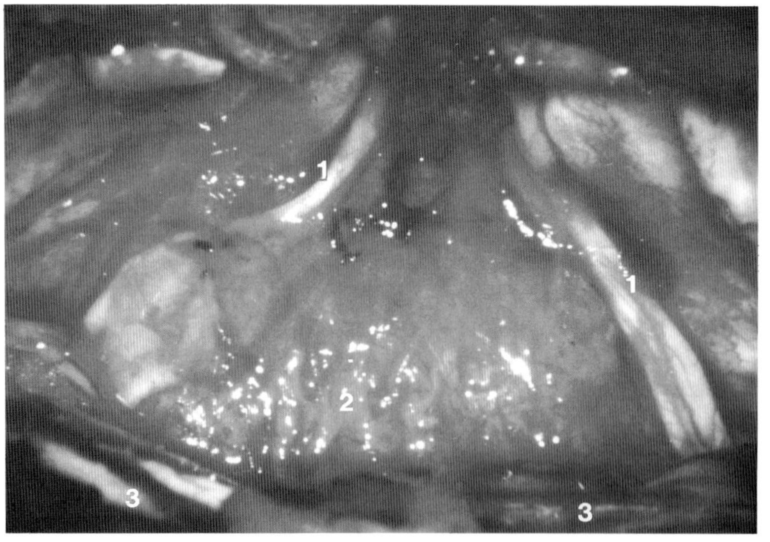

Fig. 4.4. Intraoperative exposure of a suprasellar meningioma through a bifrontal craniotomy. *1*, Olfactory tract; *2*, tumor; *3*, retractor on the frontal lobes

the A1 segment, and from the perforating branches arising from both the anterior communicating artery and the A1 segment. These perforators supply the septum pellucidum, medial portion of the anterior commissure, pillars of the fornix, optic chiasm, paraolfactory area, anterior limb of the internal capsule, anteroinferior part of the striatum, anterior hypothalamus (A1 branches), infundibulum, optic chiasm subcallosal, and preoptic areas of the hypothalamus (anterior communicating artery branches) [15]. It is mandatory that each arterial twig overlying the tumor be considered a perforator until it has been completely isolated and shown to enter only the tumor. Only at this time are coagulation and division of these small arteries allowed.

We perform this arterial-tumor dissection using microtumor forceps in one hand and regular microforceps in the other to pull the tumor very gently away from the vessel and, respectively, to lift the vessel off the tumor. The usefulness of a suction-irrigator device is evident at this time. The same technique is used when dealing with the optic nerves and chiasm. This separation of tumor vessel from brain is alternated with removal of the now freed bits of tumor, which may be accomplished using microscissors after coagulation of the base of the piece to be excised or using the ultrasonic aspirator. We think that the use of ultrasonic aspirator, laser, or bipolar coagulation in dealing with portions of the tumor known or presumed to be in close contact with these vital neurovascular structures is dangerous and should be discouraged. Again, the freeing of the tumor from these vital structures is greatly facilitated by the multiple ports of entry to the tumor that a bifrontal approach afford. We strongly encourage the alternate use of more than one angle of access to the tumor because that which is impossible or difficult from one angle may be easier from another. At the completion of tumor removal the dural attachment (Fig. 4.5c) is dealt in the same way as described in Chap. 3.

Fig. 4.5a–c. Intraoperative removal of suprasellar meningioma. **a, b** Tumor is being removed from the optic nerve (**a**) and chiasm (**b**). *1*, Cotton; *2*, tumor; *3*, optic nerve; *4*, planum sphenoidale; *5*, internal carotid artery; *6*, anterior angle of the optic chiasm. **c** Tumor attachment to the skull base is burred away using the diamond bit. *1*, Tumor; *2*, skull base; *3*, diamond burr

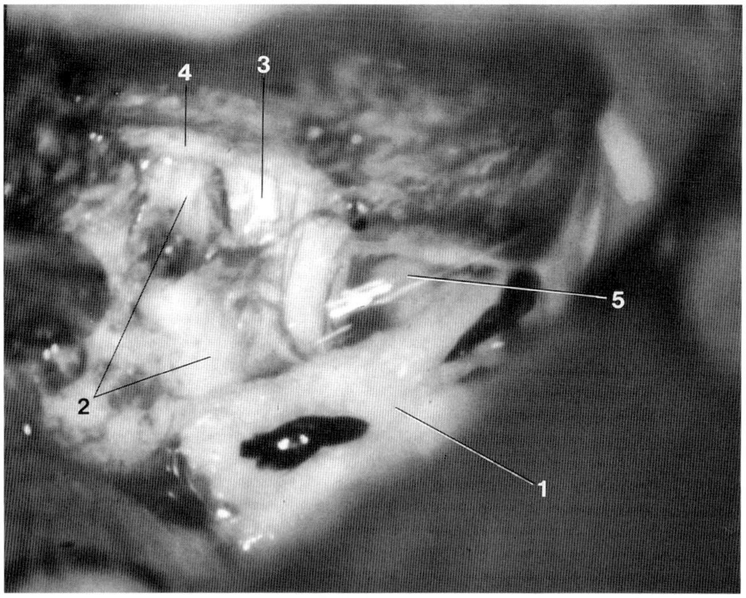

a

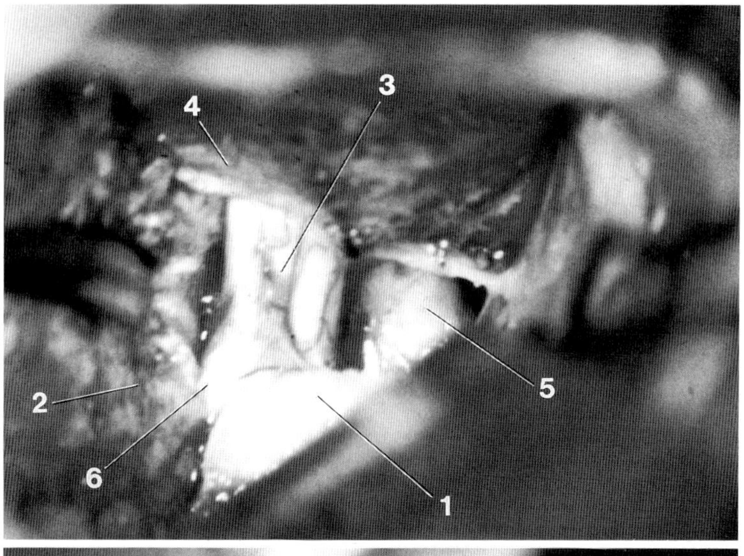

b

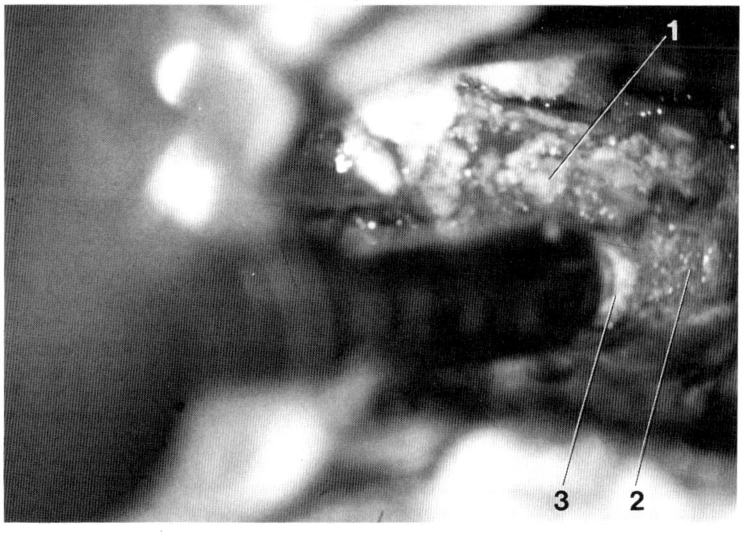

c

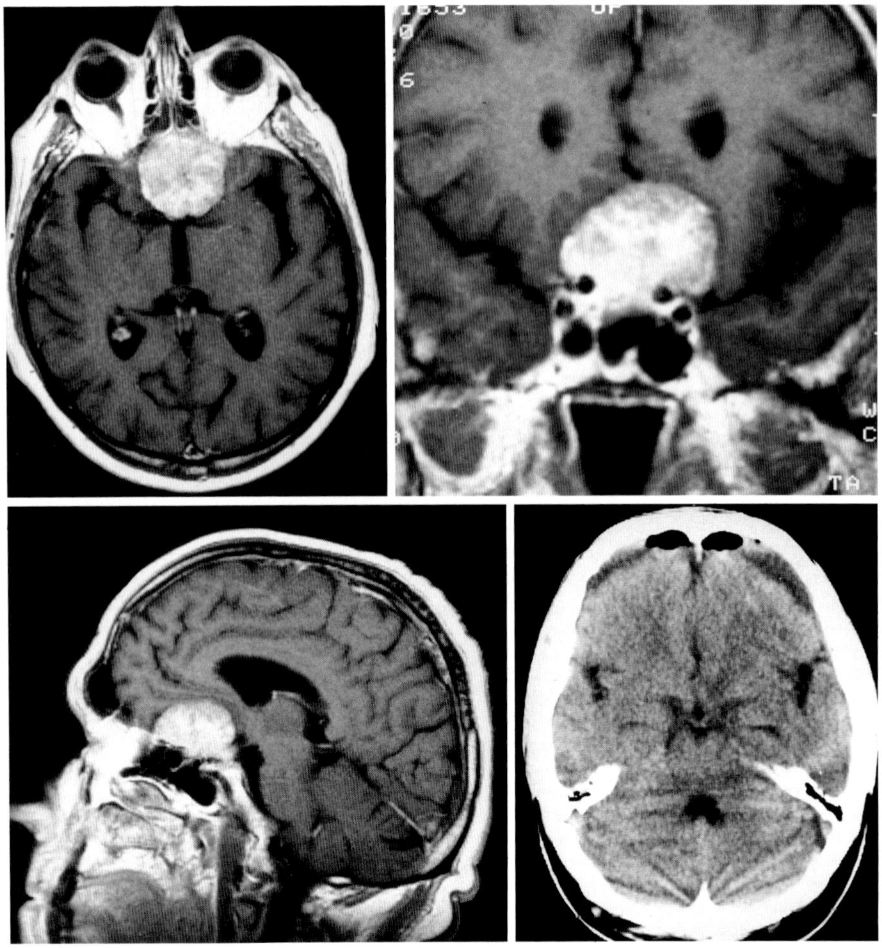

Fig. 4.6a–d. Gadolinium-enhanced axial (**a**), coronal (**b**), and sagittal (**c**) scans show a hyperintense lesion in the suprasellar area. **b** The tumor partially surrounds both supraclinoid internal carotid arteries. A tuberculum sellae meningioma was completely removed through a bifrontal craniotomy. **d** Postoperative axial CT scan shows total tumor removal

Illustrative Case

A 59-year-old woman presented to us with a few years, history of decreased vision. She had an outside CT scan showing an enhancing lesion in the suprasellar area. The neurological examination was positive for severely decreased vision in both eyes, left more than right. There was primary optic atrophy in the left eye. MRI scans confirmed the CT findings, showing an enhancing lesion in the suprasellar region (Fig. 4.6a–c). Through a bifrontal craniotomy a suprasellar tumor originating from the tuberculum sellae enveloping the supraclinoid ICA and both optic nerves and extending into the sella turcica was completely removed. The postoperative course was uncomplicated with improvement of vision on the right. Postoperative CT showed complete tumor removal (Fig. 4.6d).

References

1. Al Mefty O, Holoubi A, Rifai A, Fox JL (1985) Microsurgical removal of suprasellar meningiomas. Neurosurgery 16:364–372
2. Cushing H, Eisenhardt C (1962) Meningiomas. Their classification, regional behavior, life history and surgical end results. Hafner, New York, pp 225–241
3. Grant FC (1952) Meningioma of the tuberculum sellae. Arch Neurol Psychiatry 68:411–412
4. Gregorius FK, Hepler RS, Stern WE (1975) Loss and recovery of vision with suprasellar meningiomas. J Neurosurg 42:69–75

5. Guiot G, Derome P, Viscot A (1970) Meningeomes suprasellaires retrochiasmatiques. Neurochirurgie 16: 273–285
6. Kadis GN, Mount LA, Ganti SR (1979) The importance of early diagnosis and treatment of the meningiomas of the planum sphenoidale and tuberculum sellae: a retrospective study of 105 cases. Surg Neurol 12:367–371
7. Kempe L (1968) Operative neurosurgery, vol 1. Springer, Berlin Heidelberg New York, pp 94–97
8. Logue V (1979) Surgery of meningiomas. In: Symon L (ed) Operative surgery: neurosurgery. Butterworths, London, pp 128–173
9. MacCarty CS, Piepgras DG, Ebersold NJ (1982) Meningeal tumors of the brain. In: Youmans J (ed) Neurological surgery: a comprehensive reference guide to the diagnosis and management of neurosurgical problems, 2nd edn. Saunders, Philadelphia, pp 2936–2966
10. Morley TP (1973) Tumors of the cranial meninges. In: Youmans J (ed) Neurological surgery: a comprehensive reference guide to the diagnosis and management of neurosurgical problems, 1st edn. Saunders, Philadelphia, pp 1388–1411
11. Ojemann RG, Swann KW (1988) Surgical management of olfactory groove, suprasellar and medial sphenoid wing meningiomas. In: Schmidek HH, Sweet WH (eds) Operative neurosurgical techniques: indications, methods and results, vol 1, 2nd edn. Grune and Stratton, New York, pp 531–545
12. Rosenstein J, Symon L (1984) Surgical management of suprasellar meningioma. II. Prognosis for visual function following craniotomy. J Neurosurg 61:642–648
13. Symon L (1977) Olfactory groove and suprasellar meningiomas. In: Krayenbuhl H (ed) Advances and technical standards in neurosurgery, vol 4. Springer-Verlag, Berlin Heidelberg New York, pp 67–91
14. Symon L, Rosenstein J (1984) Surgical management of suprasellar meningioma. I. The influence of tumor size, duration of symptoms and microsurgery on surgical outcome in 101 patients. J Neurosurg 61:633–641
15. Yasargil MG (1984) Microneurosurgery, vol 1. Thieme, Stuttgart, pp 92, 108

CHAPTER 5

Medial Sphenoid Wing Meningiomas

General Considerations

Cushing was the first to systematize sphenoid wing meningiomas, dividing them into those arising from the inner third (deep, medial, or clinoidal third meningiomas), middle third (alar meningiomas), and outer third (pterional meningiomas) [3]. This distinction is still useful and practical today, not only because the respective symptoms differ, but also because the surgical problems, strategies, and goals vary greatly from one region to another. Clinoidal sphenoidal wing meningiomas grow mainly into the middle fossa and parasellar region. They may displace but usually surround the middle cerebral artery, supracavernous internal carotid artery, and optic nerve; the cavernous sinus may be compressed or invaded by these tumors. In large tumors the frontal and temporal lobes are compressed from below and are separated by the tumor. The symptoms associated with this type of tumor growth consist mainly of visual disturbances in the form of decreased vision homolaterally and visual field defect due to compression of the lateral chiasm and proximal optic tract; seizures may also occur [2]. Some tumors have an en plaque type of growth with diffuse infiltration of the dura and bone of the inner middle fossa and posterior frontal fossa. This type of tumor commonly invades the cavernous sinus, optic foramen, superior orbital fissure, orbit, greater and lesser wings of the sphenoid, and occasionally the body of the sphenoid and sphenoid sinus; through massive bony invasion or via the middle fossa foramina it may reach the pterygopalatine and infratemporal fossa. This type of tumor may present with proptosis (orbital outflow congestion, orbital tumor, hyperostosis), extraocular movement imbalances, facial pain, or visual disturbances [2]. Mixed forms also exist [2].

CT scans show an homogeneously enhancing mass in the medial sphenoid ridge area extending into the temporal and, at least with large tumors, in the frontal fossa. Extension of the mass into the orbit and paranasal sinuses is also well depicted. Due to the propensity of this tumor to invade the bone, a detailed bony study of the orbital roof, superior orbital fissure, sphenoid bone and petrous apex area is recommended (Fig. 5.1). MRI scans show the relationship between tumor and blood vessels better than do CT scans. Angiography typically shows elevation of the middle cerebral artery and of the supraclinoidal internal carotid artery which may be medially displaced. If the tumor invades the cavernous sinus, there may be narrowing of the intracavernous internal carotid artery. En plaque tumor may show less mass effect, a marked vascular stain in the medial middle fossa together with pronounced encasement and narrowing of the intracavernous and supraclinoidal internal carotid artery (Fig. 5.2).

Personal Series

Our clinical material is presented in Table 5.1. Decreased vision was the most common presenting symptom; exophthalmus was also quite common. While presence of V 1 disturbance could be seen in still circumscribed tumors, involvement of V 2 and even more so V 3 indicated cavernous sinus involvement or diffuse dural invasion. The cavernous sinus was seen to be involved at surgery 12 times, and in only 3 cases was its involvement not associated with massive dural invasion. Of the four deaths one was from massive pulmonary emboli 2 days after an uneventful postoperative recovery; two patients died of diencephalic injury without having regained

5.1

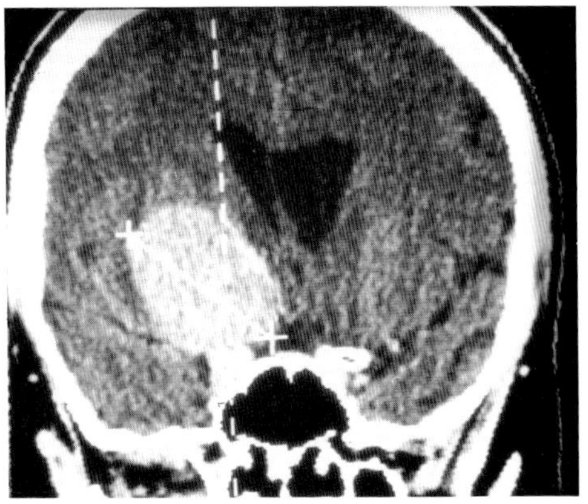

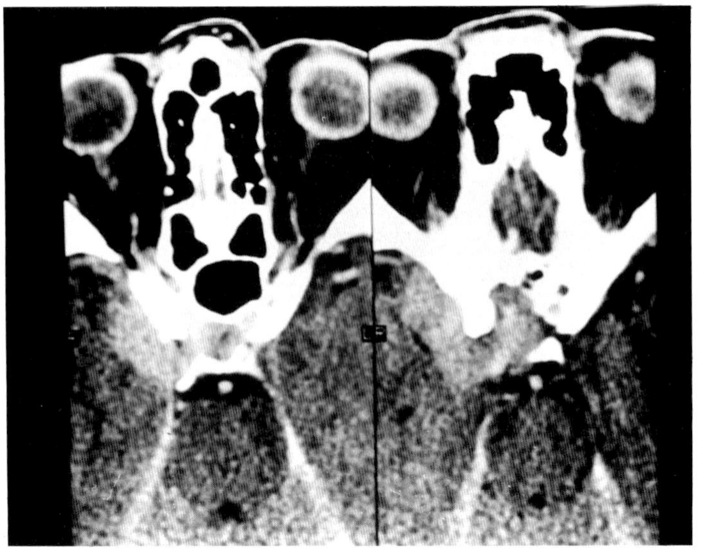

5.2

Fig. 5.1. Typical CT appearance of a globular en masse medial sphenoid wing meningioma

Fig. 5.2. CT scan of an en plaque medial sphenoid wing meningioma. The orbit, sella turcica, and tickened sphenoid bone are invaded by the tumor

Table 5.1 Medial sphenoid wing meningiomas

Number	27
Age: range/mean/median (years)	22 – 80/58/55
Women/men	20/7
Symptom (most common)	Decreased vision
Sign (most common)	Decreased visus
Tumor removal	
Total	18
Subtotal	9
Outcome	
Good	17
Fair	4
Poor	2
Deaths	4

consciousness, and the fourth died, 2 days after an uneventful postoperative recovery, of a massive intracerebral hemorrhage probably due to a surgical vascular lesion. In each a complete removal had been judged to be accomplished at surgery; autopsy showed that only one patient had residual tumor. The two poor outcomes were the result of aphasia and severe hemiparesis. In four patients the visual function deteriorated postoperatively while in 17 it was unchanged or improved.

Surgical Considerations

The goals of surgery in medial sphenoid wing meningiomas depend on the type of tumor growth. Tumors that grow in a globular fashion with a relatively well-defined point of origin on the medial sphenoid wing if completely removed carry the same good clinical prognosis of meningiomas arising elsewhere. However, their complete surgical removal may represent a formidable task due to the tight encasement of the internal carotid artery and its branches by the tumor lobules. Surgical judgement must therefore be exercised on a case-by-case basis, taking into account, among other variables, the patient's age and symptoms in deciding whether to pursue a radical excision with its attending risks. On the other hand, we believe that en plaque meningiomas of the medial middle fossa are not amenable to a surgical cure due to their diffuse invasion of the basal dura, cavernous sinus, bone, and vascular and neural foramina of the medial middle fossa. The goal of surgery in these cases should be the cautious removal of whatever globular part of the tumor exists, together with specific surgical measures aimed at relieving the patient's symptoms. A wide orbital decompression with intraorbital tumor removal may be indicated to relieve proptosis or optic nerve compression, while decompression of the trigeminal branches may be performed to relieve facial pain; radiation therapy is then recommended in the hope of halting tumor progression. We believe that inflicting to the patients any unnecessary morbidity or, worse, mortality in a futile attempt to "completely" remove a lesion that is not surgically completely removable must be rejected.

Cushing approached these tumors using a wide unilateral frontal craniotomy with removal of the anterior frontal lobe [3]. Ojemann [9], Kempe [5], McCarty [7], and Bonnal [1] use a frontotemporal craniotomy with opening of the medial sylvian fissure, retraction of frontal and temporal lobes, and an attack on the tumor following the lesser sphenoid wing. At times Bonnal [1] performs a second procedure to remove the tumor in the craniofacial cavities according to the technique of Derome and Guiot [4]. Morley recommends an extended frontotemporal craniotomy with amputation of the temporal pole [8], while Logue resects the inferolateral frontal lobe [6]. We approach these tumors through a frontotemporal craniotomy placed on the side of the tumor. The surgical technique is the following (see Figs. 5.3–5.8).

Position. The patient is placed supine with the head slightly elevated above the level of the heart, rotated approximately 60° toward the contralateral side, so as to bring the malar eminence to the uppermost portion of the field.

Scalp Flap. The skin incision begins just above the zygoma and just in front of the tragus, avoiding the main trunk of the superficial temporal artery, goes vertically superiorly crossing the superior temporal line and then curves anteriorly and superiorly to end 2 cm from the midline of the frontal region just behind the hairline (Fig. 5.3). The scalp flap is then separated from the underlying temporal fascia and inferiorly retracted. The temporal muscle is incised at the anterior and posterior end of the exposed field, separated from the bone and retracted inferiorly.

Craniotomy. The bone is exposed down to the frontozygomatic suture anteriorly and 1–2 cm in front of the root of the zygomatic arch posteriorly. The exposure includes the zygomatic portion of the frontal bone, the greater wing of the sphenoid, the anterior portion of the temporal squama and corresponding lateral portions of the frontal and parietal bone. The first burrhole is placed just above

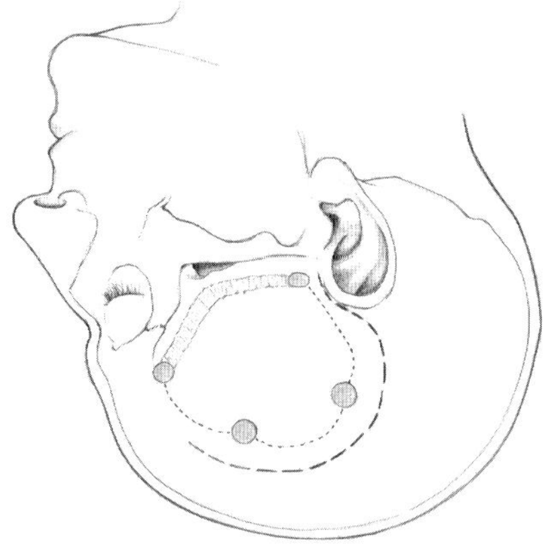

Fig. 5.3. Skin incision and bone flap

the frontozygomatic suture; it is directed superiorly and posteriorly and gives access to the posterolateral corner of the frontal fossa. This is the keyhole and the same precautions described in Chap. 3 apply to its execution. A second burrhole is placed in the frontal bone 4 cm superior to the first; a third burrhole is in the parietal bone behind the coronal suture and along the superior temporal line. The last burrhole is placed in the temporal squama about 4 cm behind the first one (Fig. 5.3). If access to the middle temporal lobe is desired, the fourth burrhole must be in the temporal squama above the root of the zygomatic arch; this requires that the skin flap swing more posteriorly, reaching the posterior aspect of the pinna. The burrholes are then connected using a craniotome. It may be advisable for cosmetic reasons to connect the first and second burrholes with a Gigli saw that yields a thinner cut than the craniotome. The second and third and the third and fourth burrholes are then connected using a craniotome. The bone between the first and fourth burrholes is then rongeured away or drilled off, reaching the greater wing of the sphenoid from both sides. At this level the flap is gently fractured, and it is hinged on the already dissected temporal muscle (Fig. 5.4). The greater wing of the sphenoid and the temporal squama are then rongeured away to the horizontal portion of the skull base. At this point and before opening of the dura, tenting sutures are inserted to avoid oozing into the field and to prevent intraoperative epidural clot due to sudden decrease in brain volume.

Dura Opening. The dura is opened in a trap-door fashion crossing the sylvian fissure, exposing the

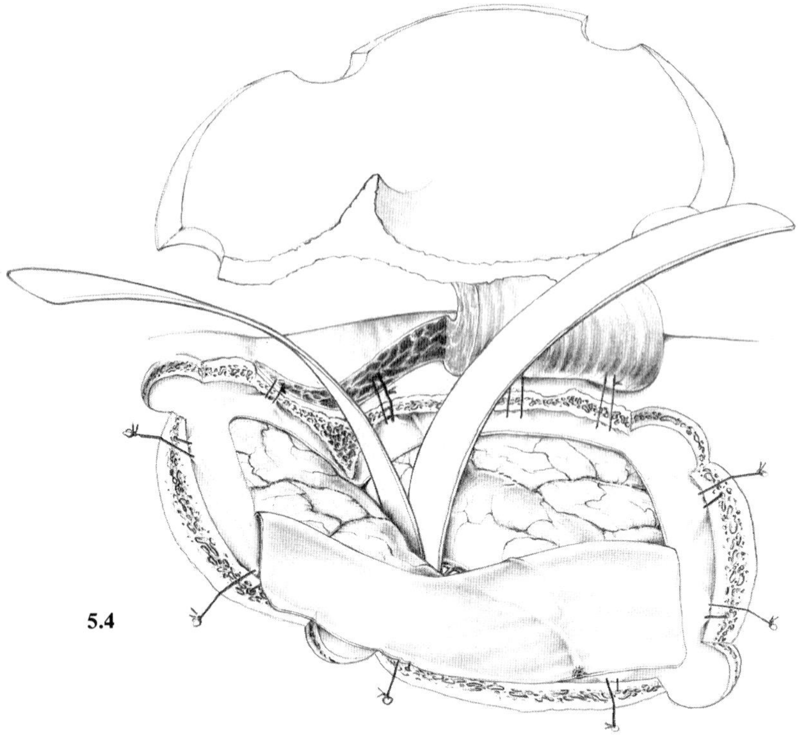

5.4

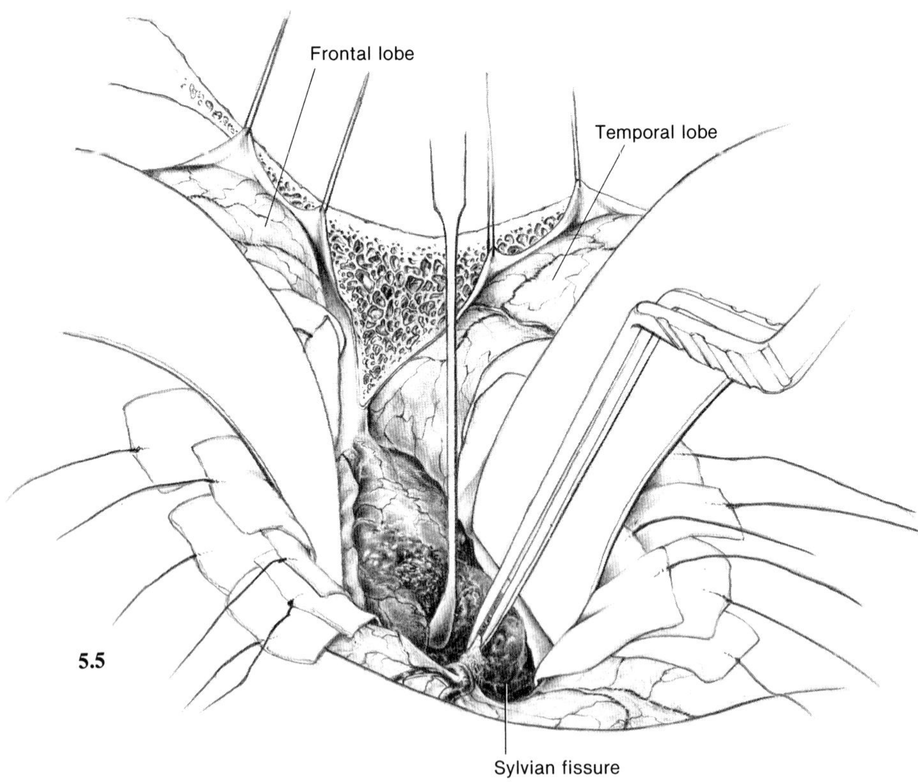

5.5

Fig. 5.4. After a frontotemporal craniotomy, the dura is opened in a trap-door fashion, and the tumor is approached through the sylvian fissure

Fig. 5.5. The tumor is visualized laterally from above and resected in a piecemeal fashion with the aid of bipolar forceps

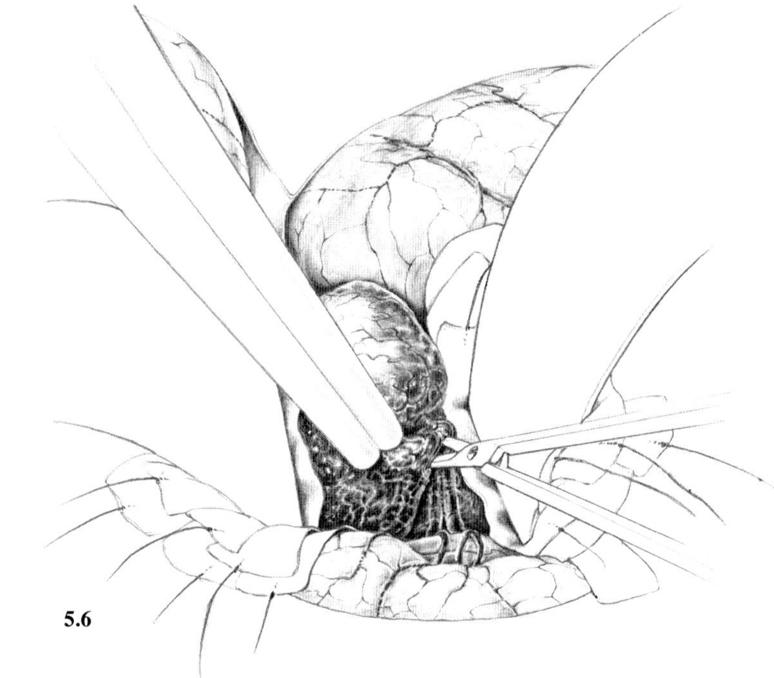

5.6

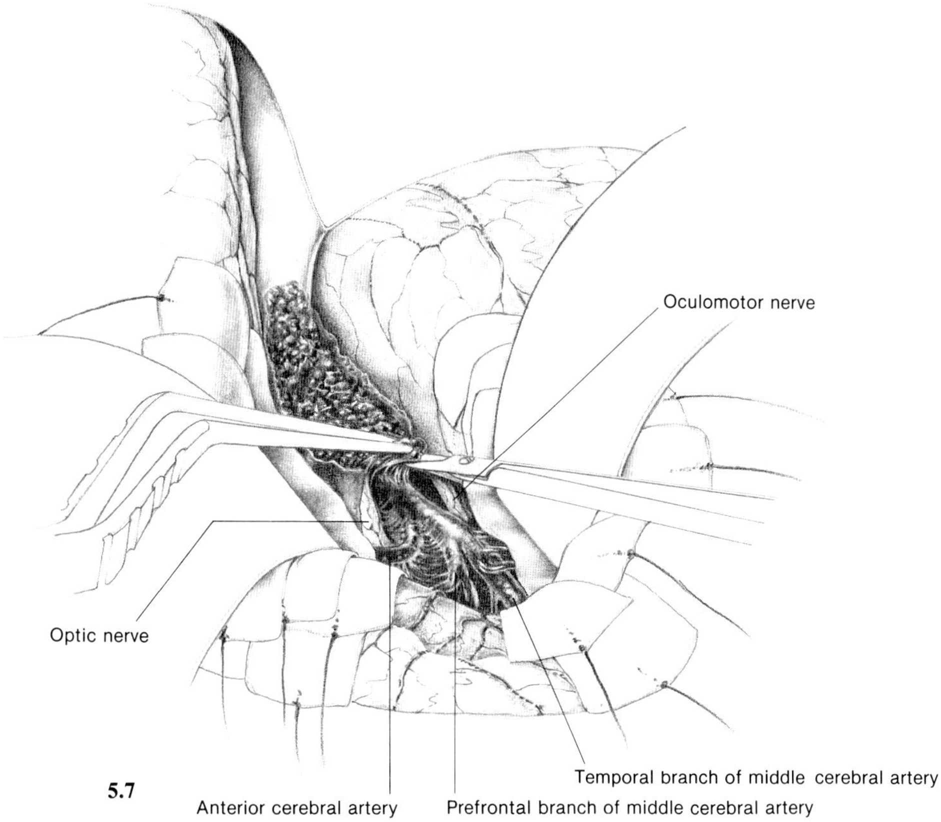

5.7

Fig. 5.6. The tumor capsule is separated from the middle cerebral artery

Fig. 5.7. The resection continues along the middle cerebral artery to the internal carotid

Table 6.1. Middle sphenoid wing meningiomas

Number	18
Age: range/mean/median (years)	27–75/48/51.5
Women/men	15/3
Symptom (most common)	Bulging of the eye
Sign (most common)	Exophthalmos
Tumor removal	
Total	18
Subtotal	0
Outcome	
Good	18
Fair	0
Poor	0
Deaths	0

and negative results on neurological examination. There was one patient with bilateral middle sphenoid wing meningioma. The tumor was completely removed in each patient, and each had a good outcome.

Illustrative Case

A 79-year-old woman presented to us with 4 years' history of headache and with right-sided weakness of a few weeks' duration. CT scans showed a large meningioma occupying the middle cranial fossa (Fig. 6.1 a, b). At surgery a large meningioma originating from the middle portion of the sphenoid wing was completely removed (Fig. 6.1 c). Postoperatively she had increased right-sided weakness and mild aphasia that completely resolved in 6 months.

Reference

1. Cushing H, Eisenhardt C (1962) Meningiomas. Their classification, regional behavior, life history and surgical end results. Hafner, New York, pp 320–342

CHAPTER 7

Lateral Sphenoid Wing Meningiomas

General Considerations

Lateral sphenoid wing meningiomas may exhibit two patterns of growth. One is globular, and a tumor showing this type of growth is, from a surgical standpoint, a low convexity meningioma, which is not discussed here further. The other is an en plaque type of growth, almost invariably with diffuse bone and dural invasion. These tumors tend to have a small intradural component, a wide dural component, and an even wider bony extension. As noted by Cushing, they tend to invade the greater wing of the sphenoid both in its lateral component, that is, the posterior portion of the lateral orbital wall, and in its medial component, the anterior portion of the middle cranial fossa and the posterior orbital wall [2]. It can be seen that they may invade the orbit both from its posterior and from its lateral wall. Their orbital invasion may be confined to the periorbita, representing the continuation of the outer dural layer, or extend to the dural layer of the optic nerve, representing the continuation of the inner part of the dura. Once such an event takes place, the tumor may grow into the orbital content (orbital fat, orbital muscle, orbital nerves), including the optic nerve where the tumor may grow intra- and/or extradurally. Continuing in its medial invasion the tumor may invade the cavernous sinus dura and grow inside the cavernous sinus cavity, while through the middle fossa foramina (rotundum, ovale, spinosum) the tumor may reach the pterygopalatine and infratemporal fossa. The pterygopalatine fossa may be also invaded through the orbita, via the inferior orbital fissure, and both fossae may also be invaded by direct tumor penetration of the greater wing of the sphenoid. As noted by Cushing [2], invasion of the orbital roof (lesser wing of the sphenoid and orbital portion of the frontal bone), while possible, is not as frequent as the other pathways of spread. This type of tumor seems to represent a disease of the greater wing of the sphenoid, and this may have something to do with its abundant vascularization, the thickness of the dura, and the abundance of the arachnoid villi that are present in this area [2].

Patients usually present with exophthalmos of many years' duration, with swelling over the anterior temporal region and some degree of visual impairment [1, 3]. These symptoms are readily explained, considering the pattern of growth of the tumors with their resulting encroachment on the orbit and on the optic nerve. CT scans using bony algorithms are very useful to demonstrate the extent of the disease (see Fig. 7.2).

Personal Series

Many patients presented with headache, and all patients with hyperostosing tumors presented with exophthalmos and ocular pain. Of the four hyperostosing tumors, total tumor removal was felt to be accomplished in only one patient. All patients had a good outcome (Table 7.1).

Table 7.1. Lateral sphenoid wing meningiomas

Number	8
Age: range/mean/median (years)	46–67/57/57
Women/men	5/3
Symptom (most common)	Headache
Sign (most common)	None
Tumor removal	
Total	5
Subtotal	3
Outcome	
Good	8
Fair	0
Poor	0
Deaths	0

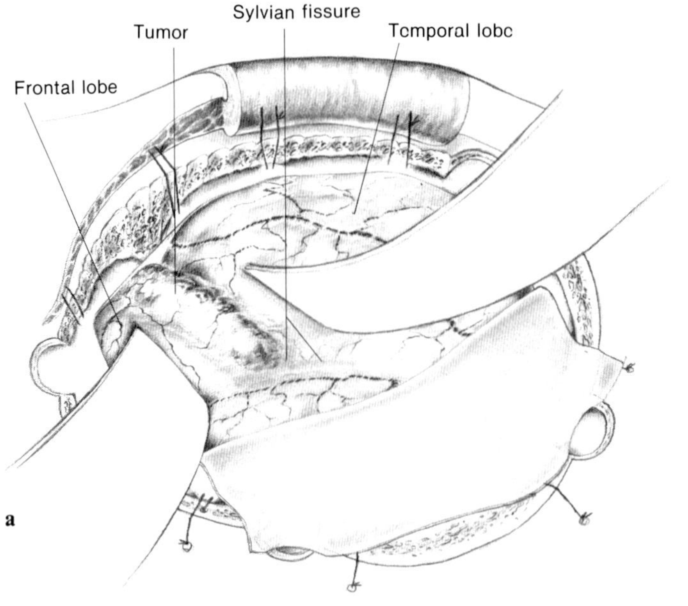

a

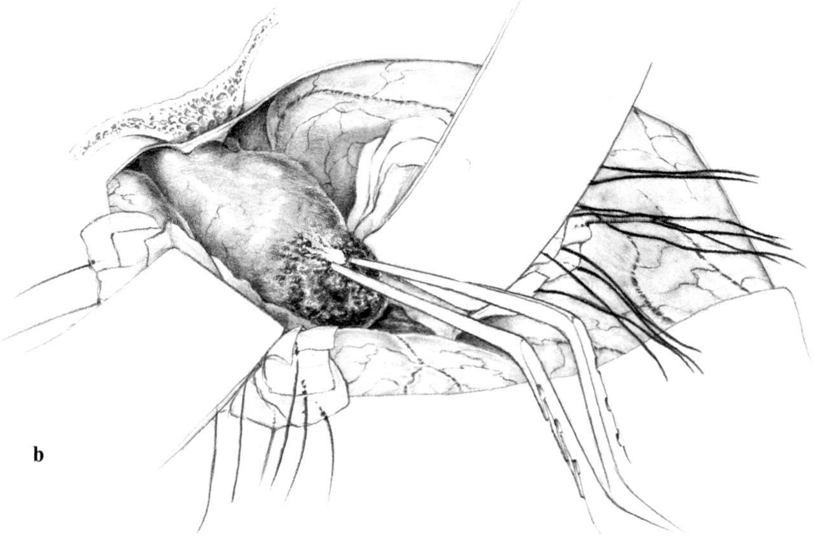

b

Fig. 7.1 a–c. Drawing of surgical steps in the removal of a lateral sphenoid wing meningioma. **a** After frontotemporal craniotomy the sylvian fissure is opened microsurgically, and the frontal and temporal lobes are retracted to expose the tumor on the lesser sphenoid wing. **b** Piecemeal tumor resection is alternated with bipolar coagulation. **c** Most of the lesser wing of the sphenoid is removed with the area of tumor attachment to ensure a complete resection

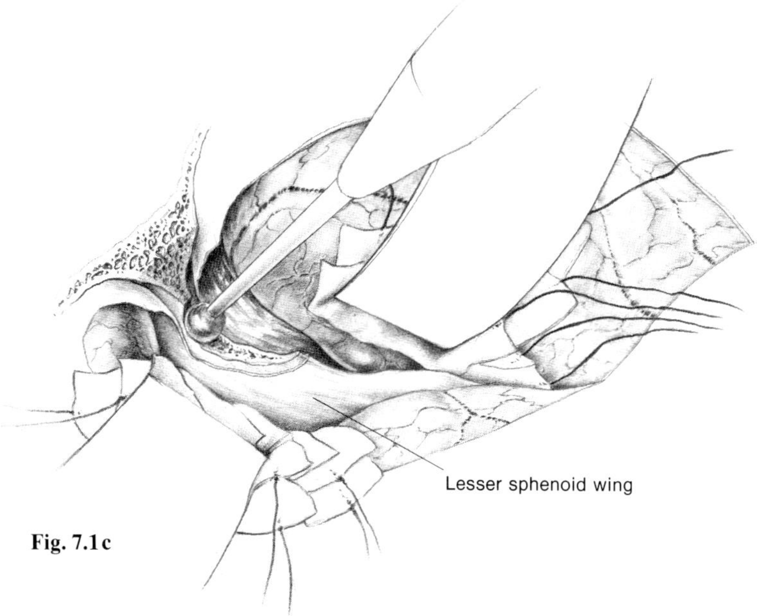

Fig. 7.1c

Surgical Considerations

Those tumors exhibiting the globular type of growth may be easily and completely removed using a pterional craniotomy (Fig. 7.1). However, we believe that those tumors showing an en plaque type of growth are – as all en plaque meningiomas – not amenable to surgical cure. Consequently the goal of surgery should be relief of the patient's symptoms; in the majority of cases this means treatment of the proptosis and decompression of the optic nerve. These surgical measures may relieve the patient's symptoms for many years. As the disease is mainly one of the greater sphenoid wing, a frontotemporal craniotomy extending as low as the zygomatic arch is recommended. If access to the infratemporal fossa is desired, the zygomatic arch may be cut and then reconstructed at the end of the procedure. A frontotemporal flap encircling the tumor is then turned, if possible: alternatively, the involved bone can be removed using a high-speed drill. Regardless of whether a flap has been turned, the next step is to remove the involved greater wing of the sphenoid, in both its lateral and medial extents. This is accomplished using a high-speed drill, and bone bleeding may be considerable. In doing so one enters the orbital cavity, taking care not to enter the periorbita, and exposes the frontal and temporal dura. If the optic nerve canal and orbital roof need to be decompressed, this is performed, again, extradurally using the high-speed drill. At this stage it may be wise to open the dura and to remove the intradural part of the tumor. Once the dura is closed, the periorbita may be opened and the intraorbital tumor removed. Great care is necessary at this stage of the operation not to injure functioning intraorbital structures (nerves and muscles). Considering that these tumors are usually not curable by surgery, we do not recommend extending the surgery beyond that which is necessary to relieve the patient's symptoms or beyond the bulk of the tumor that may be easily removable. Extensive surgery results in high risk to the patients, increased morbidity, and nevertheless no cure.

Illustrative Case

A 50-year-old woman presented to us with a 1-year history of left-sided exophthalmus and suprazygomatic fullness (Fig. 7.2a). Neurological examination was positive for a slight left VI nerve paresis. CT scans and angiography demonstrated a large hypervascular tumor extending from the temporal fossa to the cavernous sinus and invading the greater and lesser sphenoid wings (Fig. 7.2b–d). At surgery a large meningioma invading the temporal

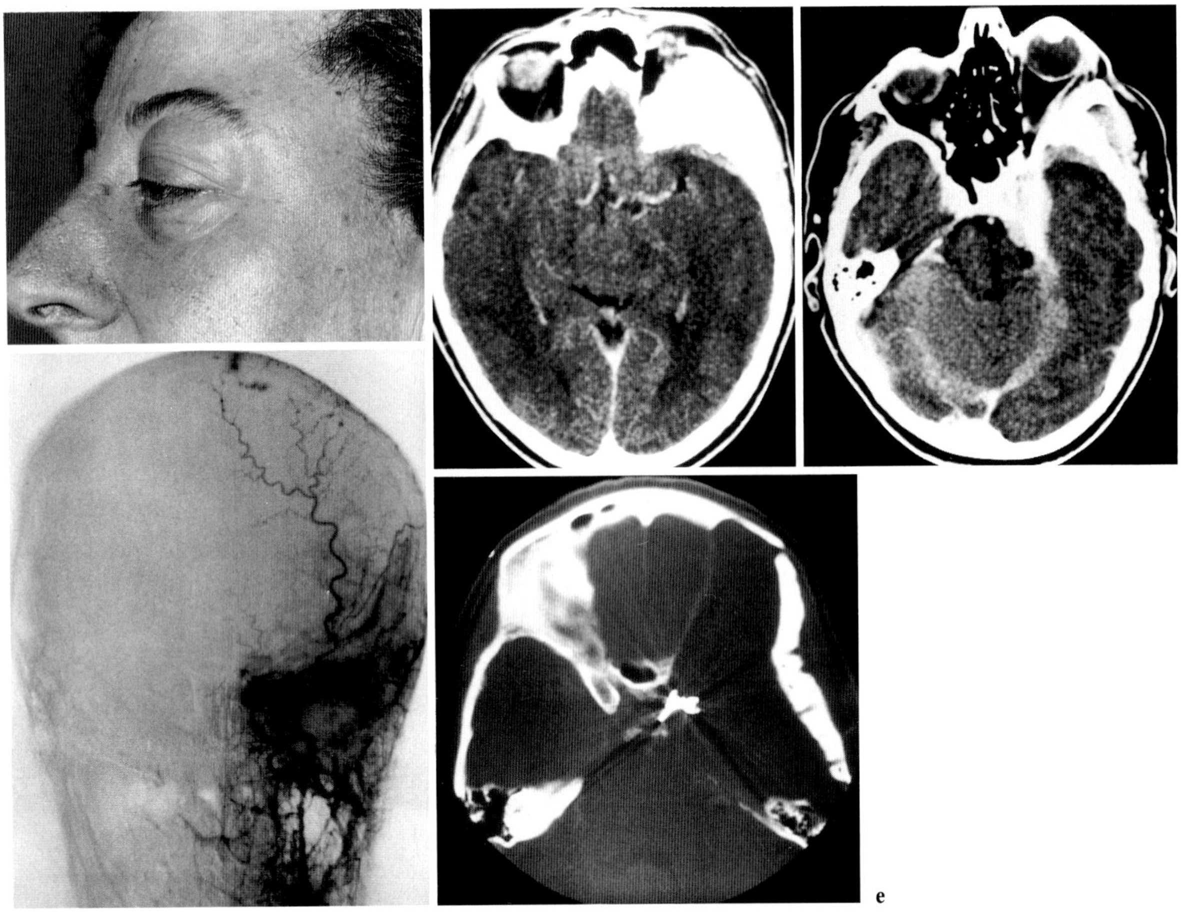

Fig. 7.2 a–e. Extensive en plaque meningioma invading the greater and lesser wing of the sphenoid, temporal fossa, cavernous sinus, and clivus. **a** The suprazygomatic and orbital fullness is evident. **b, c** CT scans show the extensive bony hyperostosis and the small soft tissue tumor component, involving the sphenoid wing, clinoid process, cavernous sinus, orbital cavity, and temporal fossa. **d** Angiogram shows the tumor stain. **e** Postoperative CT scan shows tumor removal and bony reconstruction using methylmetacrylate

squama, greater and lesser wings of the sphenoid, cavernous sinus, and clivus was radically removed. The temporal squama and orbit were reconstructed using methylmetacrylate (Fig. 7.2e). The postoperative course was uneventful, with reduction of the exophthalmus.

References

1. Bonnal J, Thibaut A, Brotchi J, Born J (1980) Invading meningiomas of the sphenoid ridge. J Neurosurg 53: 587–594
2. Cushing H, Eisenhardt C (1962) Meningiomas. Their classification, regional behavior, life history and surgical end results. Hafner, New York, pp 320–342
3. Ojemann RG (1985) Clinical features and management of meningiomas. In: Wilkins RH, Rengachary SS (eds) Neurosurgery, vol 1. McGraw-Hill, New York, pp 635–654

CHAPTER 8

The Problem of Classifying Meningiomas of the Posterior Fossa Skull Base

The surgical problems posed by meningiomas in the posterior fossa skull base depend more on their topographical location in relation to the skull base and the tentorium than on their point of dural attachment; their topographical location is a function of their direction of growth. A meningioma presenting mainly in the region corresponding to the anterior part of the posterior aspect of the petrous pyramid poses essentially the same surgical problems regardless of whether it arises from the undersurface of the anterior portion of the tent, from the posterior surface of the pyramid per se, or even from the clivus. These problems are quite different from those encountered with meningiomas presenting mainly in the posterior portion of the posterior pyramid, and both are different from those associated with incisural or petroclival meningiomas. As all these tumors can be attacked surgically at present, it is imperative in order to compare series that they be described in terms of their main topographical location (as demonstrated by CT and MRI) rather than in terms of their dural attachment.

While we are well aware of the taxonomic limitations, especially when dealing with tumors that often do not respect fixed anatomical boundaries, we propose to classify meningiomas of the posterior fossa skull base into jugular foramen, clivus, posterior pyramid, petroclival, and incisural meningiomas. Furthermore, the category of clivus meningiomas needs to be subdivided into those involving the lower clivus and foramen magnum region (craniospinal meningiomas) and those of the upper clivus. Similarly, posterior pyramid meningiomas should be divided into those located anterior as opposed to those located posterior to the internal auditory meatus. Meningiomas of the cerebellar convexity, irrespective of their point of origin on the tentorium, are not included among skull base meningiomas; because of their superficial location their surgical problems are similar to those of cerebral convexity meningiomas.

The proposed classification is a relative one and is based on the topographical location of the main tumor bulk as assessed by CT and MRI scans; it is a surgical classification in that different surgical approaches apply to different locations. It is obviously not applicable to giant tumors growing diffusely in more than one region, although the approach to such tumors may be rationalized by combining the different surgical techniques described in approaching any individual area.

CHAPTER 9

Jugular Foramen Meningiomas

General Considerations

Jugular foramen meningiomas are extremely rare; Cushing did not mention any such isolated case [1], and there are only a few reports of meningiomas involving primarily the jugular foramen [1, 4, 7].

Personal Series

In our series there have been three patients with meningiomas involving primarily the jugular foramen (Table 9.1). Two of these had bilateral acoustic neurinomas (NF_2), and their clinical symptoms were related to this; in one of the two, the tumor was growing en plaque in the jugular foramen and was partially resected. The third patient had a tumor growing intraosseously and intradurally in the region of the jugular foramen, with invasion of the lower cranial nerves. This case is described in detail below (see "Illustrative Case").

Table 9.1. Jugular foramen meningiomas

Number	3
Age: range/mean/median (years)	18–32/26/24
Women/men	2/1
Symptom (most common)	Hoarseness
Sign (most common)	Lower cranial nerve deficit
Tumor removal	
Total	2
Subtotal	1
Outcome	
Good	3
Fair	0
Poor	0
Deaths	0

Surgical Considerations

Meningiomas involving primarily the jugular foramen may be approached through a conventional lateral suboccipital craniectomy if the tumor is exclusively intradural, or through a combined craniocervical exposure if the tumor contains an extradural infratemporal portion in addition to the posterior fossa component [6].

The steps involved in exposure a jugular foramen meningioma in the intratemporal fossa are depicted in Fig. 9.1–9.8. It should be noted that, depending on the individual situation, the suboccipital craniectomy may be more extensive or the temporal bone drilling may be more limited. The approach depicted is a modification of the one described by Fisch [2]. More exposure may be obtained sacrificing the inner ear, combining the transcochlear approach of House and Hitsbelger [3] with the infratemporal approach of Fisch [2], as proposed by Pellet with the "widened transcochlear approach to the jugular foramen" [5]. Such an extensive approach, while indicated for glomus tumors, is rarely if ever needed for neurinomas or meningiomas involving the jugular foramen extradurally.

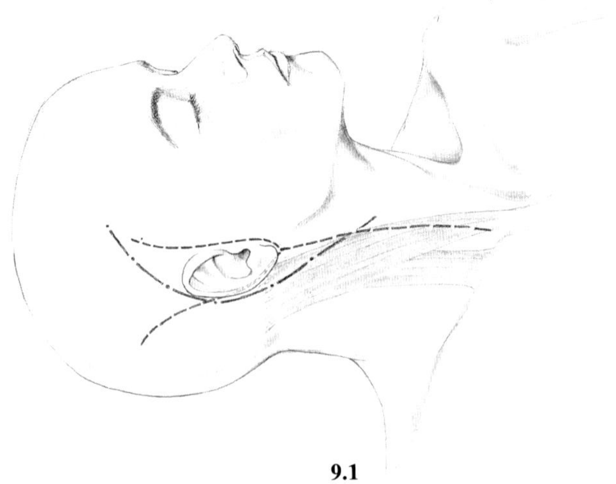

9.1

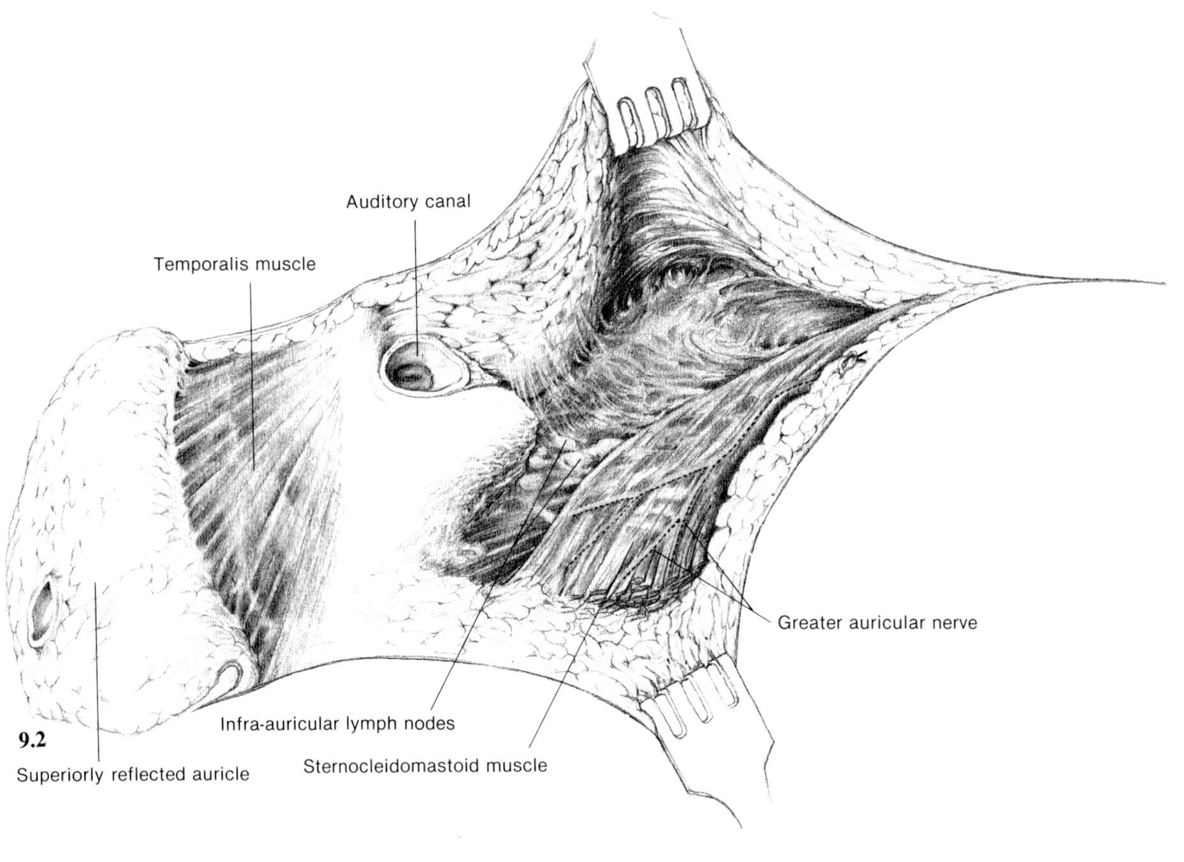
Auditory canal
Temporalis muscle
Greater auricular nerve
Infra-auricular lymph nodes
Sternocleidomastoid muscle
Superiorly reflected auricle

9.2

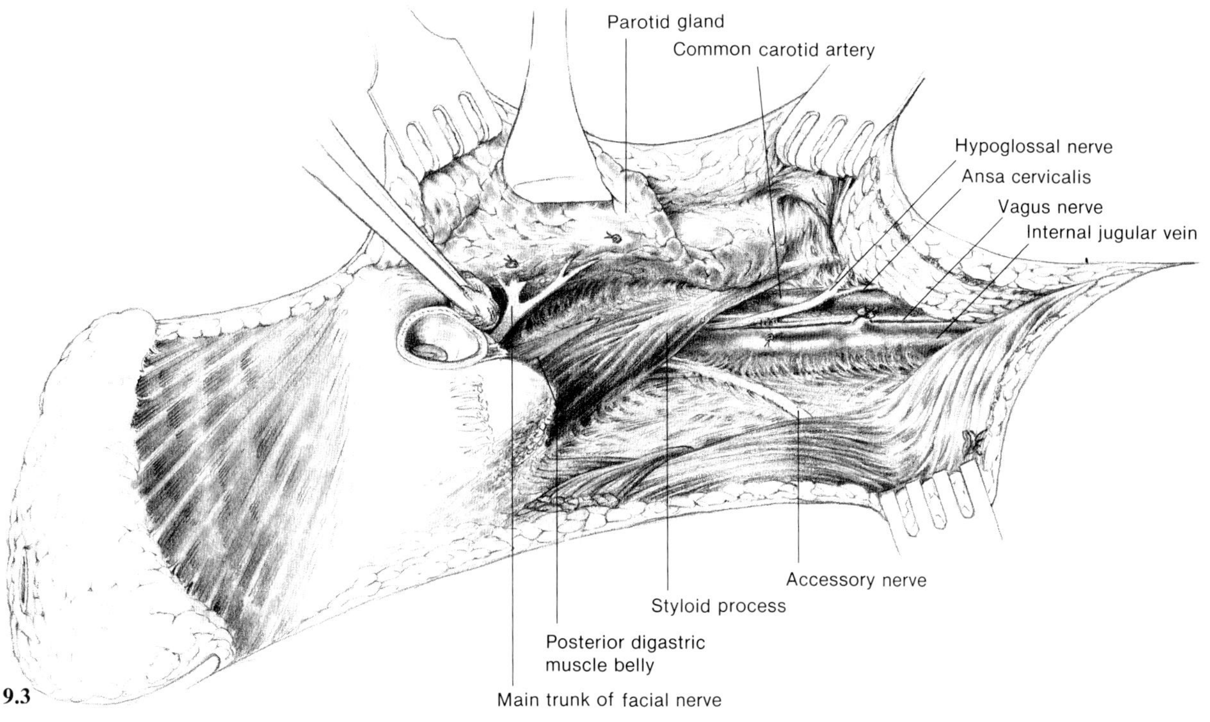

9.3

◄

Fig. 9.1. The extracranial approach to the jugular foramen. Possible skin incisions: Y-shaped incision (– – –), C-shaped incision of Fisch (– · – · – ·)

Fig. 9.2. With the Y incision, the auricle is reflected upward to expose the mastoid plane and mastoid tip, the anterior sternocleidomastoid border, and the inferior part of the parotid gland. Here the sternocleidomastoid muscle has been released from the mastoid tip and turned inferiorly, preserving its cutaneous attachment. A transparent view is given of the greater auricular nerve and its branches. Where necessary, the greater auricular nerve may be utilized as a nerve graft

▲

Fig. 9.3. Working upward from below, the surgeon exposes the accessory nerve, the neck vascular package, the vagus and hypoglossal nerves, and the posterior border of the digastric muscle. He then mobilizes the lower pole of the parotid gland. The medial point of the cartilagineous external auditory canal and the anterior border of the insertion of the sternocleidomastoid and posterior digastric muscle border serve as landmarks for locating the facial nerve. The stylomastoid foramen lies about 5 mm medial to the cartilagineous point of the auditor canal when the auricle is in its normal position. The connective tissue fibers between the cartilagineous ear canal and the parotid capsule are cleared over a wide area. The final warning sign before reaching the facial nerve is bleeding from a large arterial vessel that passes just lateral to the nerve

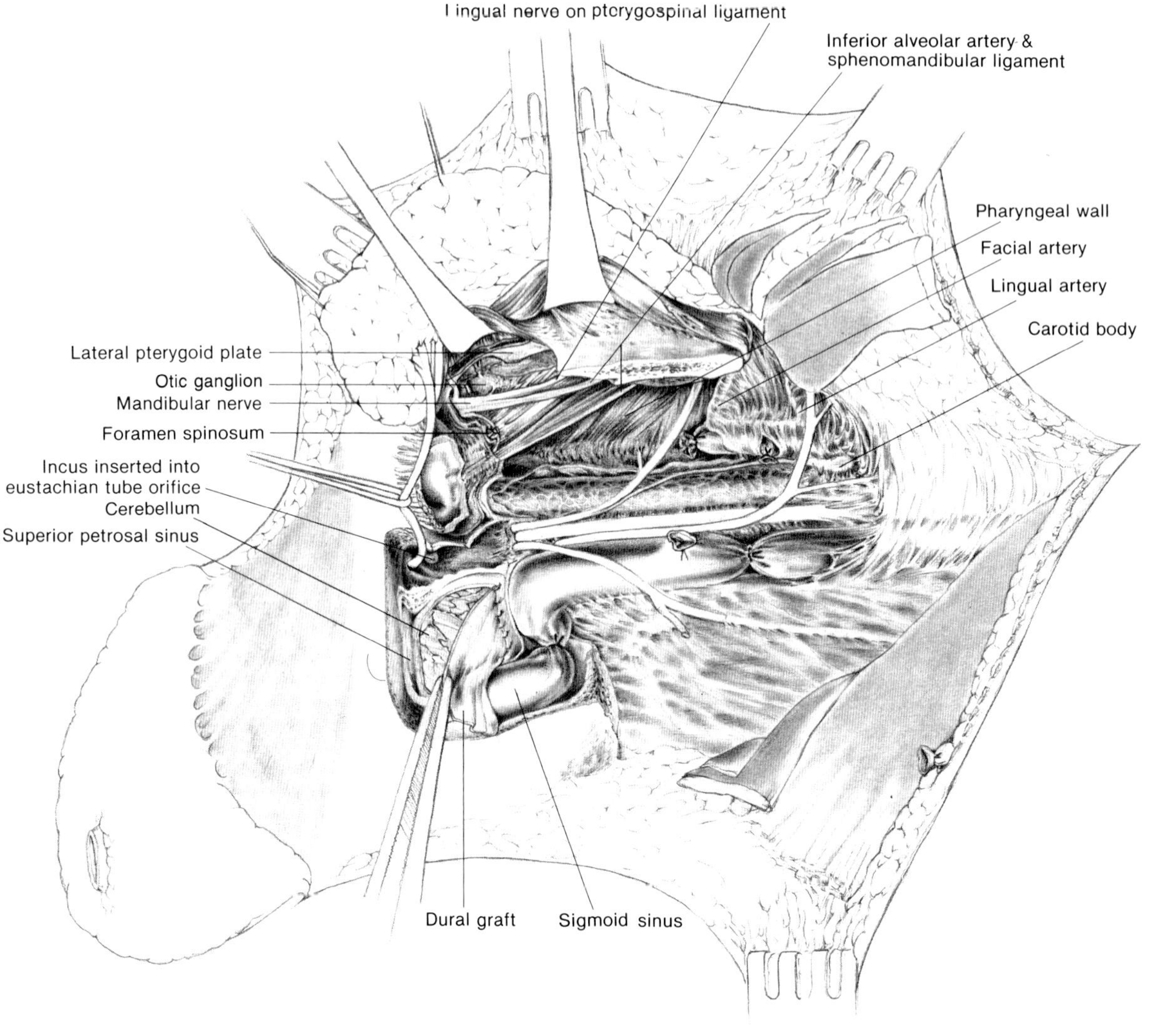

Fig. 9.7. The posteroinferior approach is extended by marginal resection of the vertical mandibular ramus giving access to the lateral middle skull base with the foramen ovale and lateral plate of the pterygoid process, and also to the lateral pharyngeal wall and the nasopharynx. Posteriorly, intracranial access can be gained by removing the dura of the posterior and middle fossae. The sigmoid sinus and internal jugular may be ligated at this stage if necessary. The dural defect is repaired with a dural graft. A partial petrosectomy may be performed

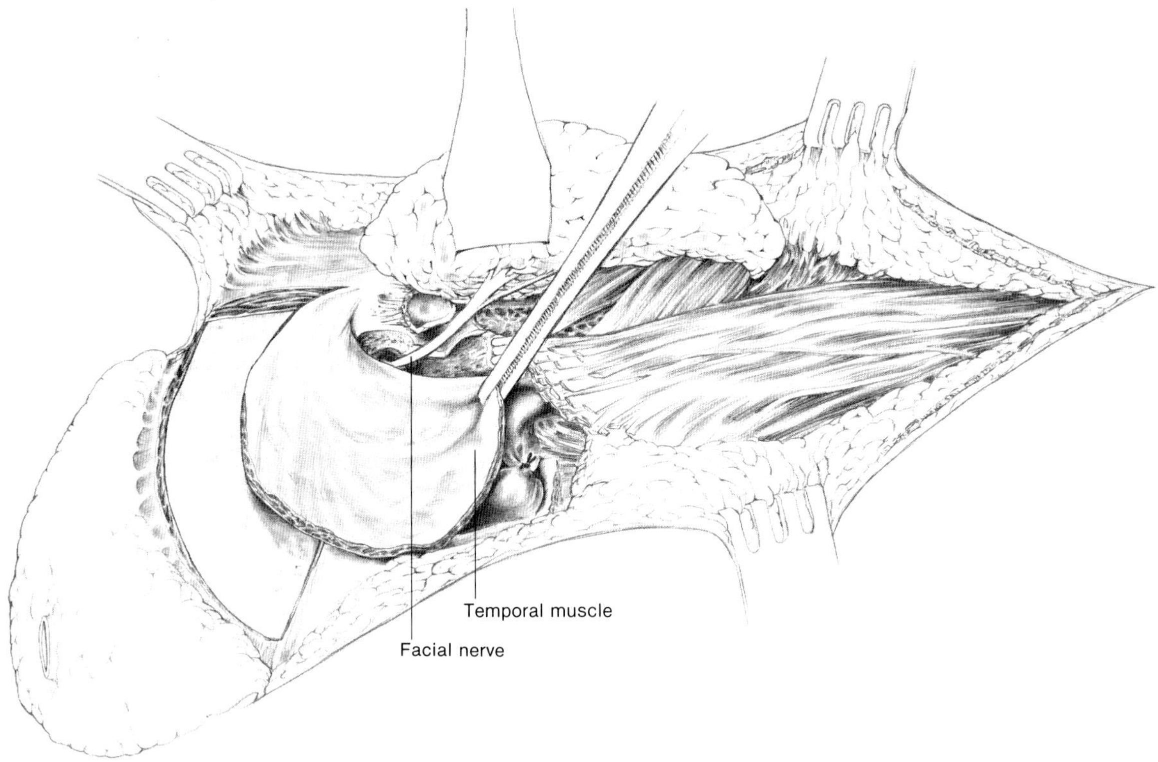

Fig. 9.8. The parotid gland is restored to its bed, and a temporal muscle flap is rotated into the field to partially restore the surgical cavity. This is done when distal release of the sternocleidomastoid muscle from the sternum and clavicle is not available for cavity ablation

Illustrative Case

A 30-year-old man presented to us with a 12-year history of hoarseness, 10-year history of right shoulder weakness, and 1-year history of decreased tongue function. The neurological examination was positive for a IX–XII cranial nerve palsy on the right side. CT scans showed a hyperostotic tumor in the region of the right jugular foramen with a soft tissue mass in the posterolateral inferior skull base (Fig. 9.9). MRI scans confirmed the presence of a mass in the right jugular foramen region.

The patient was operated on in the supine position with the head turned to the left and slightly flexed. A conventional suboccipital paramedian skin incision, 1 cm medial to the mastoid and starting 2 cm above the superior nuchal line, was extended inferiorly to about the midportion of the anterior border of the sternocleidomastoid muscle. The sternocleidomastoid as well as the splenium capitis, the posterior belly of the digastric, and the obliquus capitis superior muscles were then detached from the mastoid and from the occipital squama, thus exposing the facial nerve at the stylomastoid foramen, cranial nerves IX–XII at their point of exit from the skull, and the proximal internal jugular vein. A suboccipital craniectomy was then performed which, together with a mastoidectomy, exposed the whole length of the sigmoid sinus to the level of the jugular foramen. The posteroinferior and posterosuperior parts of the jugular foramen were found to be hyperostotic due to tumor invasion and needed to be removed using the high-speed drill. After having thus opened the jugular foramen, the jugular bulb, the distal sigmoid sinus, related dura, and the distal intracranial and proximal extracranial portions of cranial nerves IX–XII were found to be involved with tumor and needed to be excised. A cable graft using the great auricular nerve was transplanted between the proximal (intracranial) and the distal (extracranial) stumps of cranial nerve XI. The dura was closed using lyodura, secured with stitches and fibrin glue, and the resection cavity was filled with

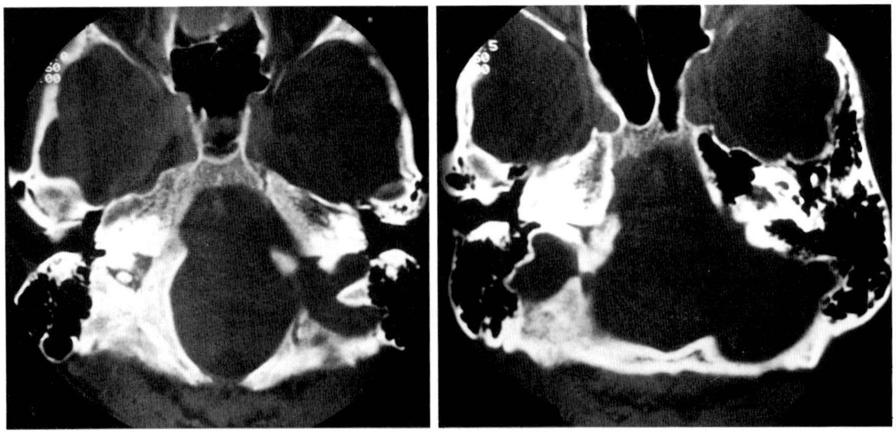

9.9a b

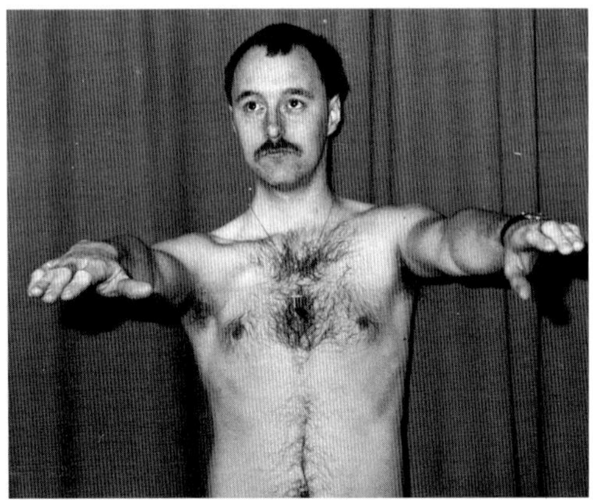

9.10

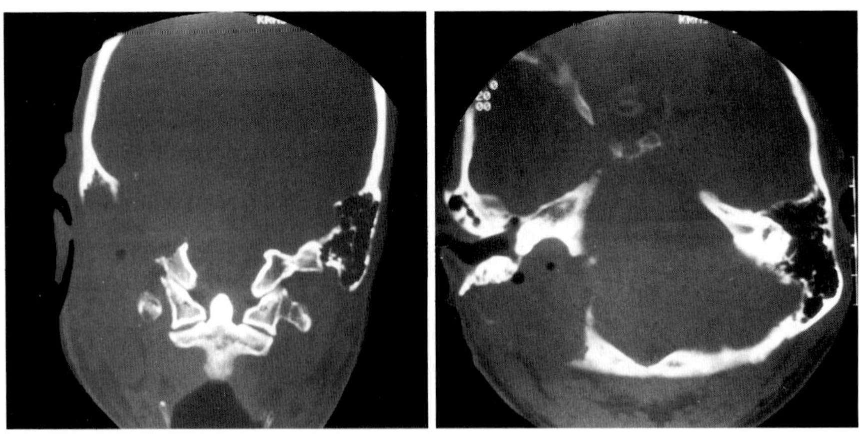

9.11a b

Fig. 9.9a, b. Preoperative CT scans show enlargement and hyperostosis of the right jugular foramen

Fig. 9.10. Postoperative picture of the patient

Fig. 9.11a, b. Postoperative coronal (**a**) and axial (**b**) CT scans show the extensive bony removal a free piece of digastric muscle. A lumbar drain was inserted and left in place for 10 days. The postoperative course was uncomplicated, and the patient was discharged with no new neurological deficit (Fig. 9.10). CT scans showing the bony removal are presented in Fig. 9.11.

References

1. Cushing H, Eisenhardt C (1962) Meningiomas. Their classification, regional behavior, life history and surgical end results. Hafner, New York
2. Fisch U, Pillsbury HC (1979) Infratemporal fossa approach to lesions in the temporal bone and base of the skull. Arch Otolaryngol Head Neck Surg 105:99–107
3. House WF, Hitselberger WE (1976) The transcochlear approach to the skull base. Arch Otolaryngol Head Neck Surg 102:334–342
4. Markham JW, Fager CA, Horrax G, Poppen JL (1955) Meningiomas of the posterior fossa. Arch Neurol Psychiatry 74:163–170
5. Pellet W, Cannoni M, Pech A (1988) The widened transcochlear approach to jugular foramen tumors. J Neurosurg 69:887–894
6. Samii M, Sepehrnia A, Mahran A, Bini W (1989) Surgery of the jugular foramen. Advances in neurosurgery. Springer, Berlin Heidelberg New York, pp 140–157
7. Yasargil MG, Mortara RW, Curcic M (1980) Meningiomas of the basal posterior cranial fossa. In: Krayenbuhl H (ed) Advances and technical standards in neurosurgery, vol 7. Springer, Berlin Heidelberg New York, pp 3–115

CHAPTER 10

Meningiomas Involving the Lower Clivus and the Foramen Magnum (Craniospinal Meningiomas)

General Considerations

Cushing divided the meningiomas involving the craniocervical junction into craniospinal and spinocranial, depending on whether the tumor was reaching the foramen magnum from above or from below. Related to this he recognized a significant surgical difference in that the craniospinal tumors were located in the cisterns anterior to the brainstem pushing the cervicomedullary junction posterolaterally while the reverse was true in spinocranial tumors [1]. According to Cushing, Hallopeau in 1872 was the first to describe a meningioma arising from the lower clivus and extending into the foramen magnum (autoptic report) [1]. Cushing himself described the case of a patient who underwent a negative cervicothoracic laminectomy with the suspicion of syringomyelia or cord glioma; autopsy disclosed a meningioma originating from the lower clivus and extending into the foramen magnum [1].

The clinical picture associated with tumors in this location is protean and unspecific, especially in the beginning. Patients may complain of vague suboccipital pain and dysesthesia in the arms. Degenerative disease of the spine is a frequent initial diagnosis [9]. By the time the patients come to surgery about 50% have weakness in the upper extremities or gait disturbances. This needs to be contrasted to the fact that almost 50% of patients have a negative neurological examination when first seen [4]. Hypoalgesia limited to the C2 dermatome, spinal accessory palsy, and bilateral stereoanesthesia of the hands, as noted by Cushing in 1938 [1], may strengthen the suspicion of a tumor localized to this area.

Personal Series

We operated on nine patients with meningiomas involving the lower clivus and the foramen magnum (craniospinal meningiomas) (Table 10.1). Weakness in the lower extremities was the most common symptom and sign. We had one patient presenting with paresis of nerves IX–XII and one patient with a syringomielic syndrome. Symptoms were usually present for 1 year, but one patient had carried the false diagnosis of cervical spondylosis for almost 10 years.

Table 10.1. Craniospinal meningiomas

Number	9
Age: range/mean/median (years)	18–72/44/54
Women/men	2/7
Symptom (most common)	Weakness of the legs
Sign (most common)	Paraparesis
Tumor removal	
Total	8
Subtotal	1
Outcome	
Good	5
Fair	3
Poor	1
Deaths	0

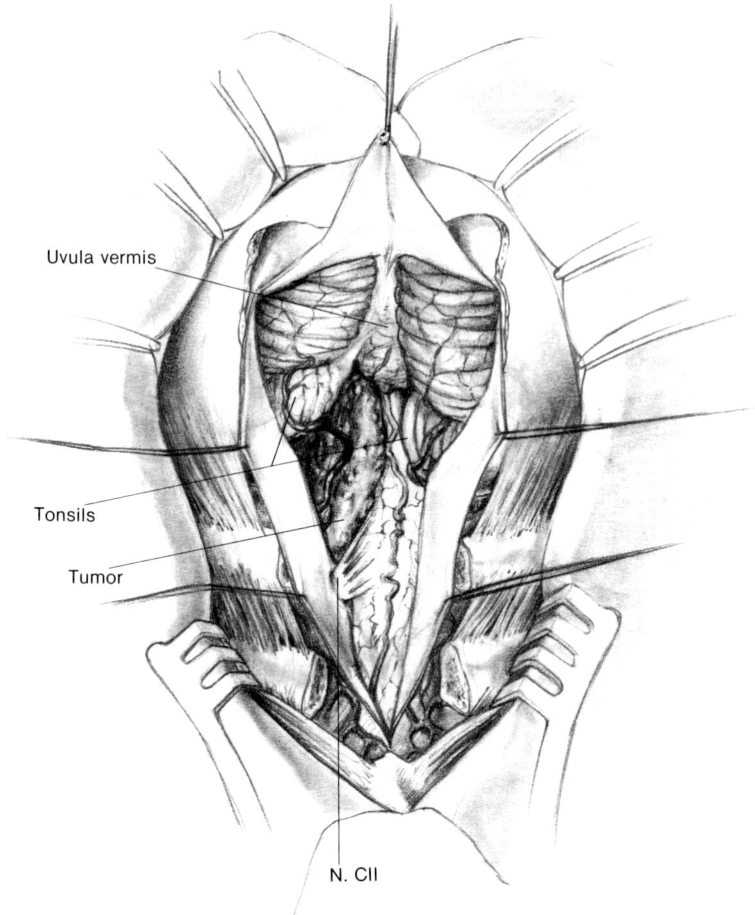

Fig. 10.3. View into the posterior cranial fossa and spinal canal after incision of the dura and retraction of its margins. The tumor presents below the left cerebellar tonsil

easier. Again, as always, judgement must be used in deciding how far it is safe to go in the individual case. While we were usually very aggressive in our own case material in dissecting the tumor from the vertebral artery, we decided not to do so in a 72-year-old woman who was operated on for syringomyelic symptoms. At the end of tumor removal the abnormal dura, usually near the intradural entrance of the vertebral artery and at the contiguous area of the hypoglossal foramen, is excised (Fig. 10.4). The dura is then closed in a watertight fashion with a continuous suture. The wound is closed in the usual way, and a compressive dressing remains in place for 5–7 days.

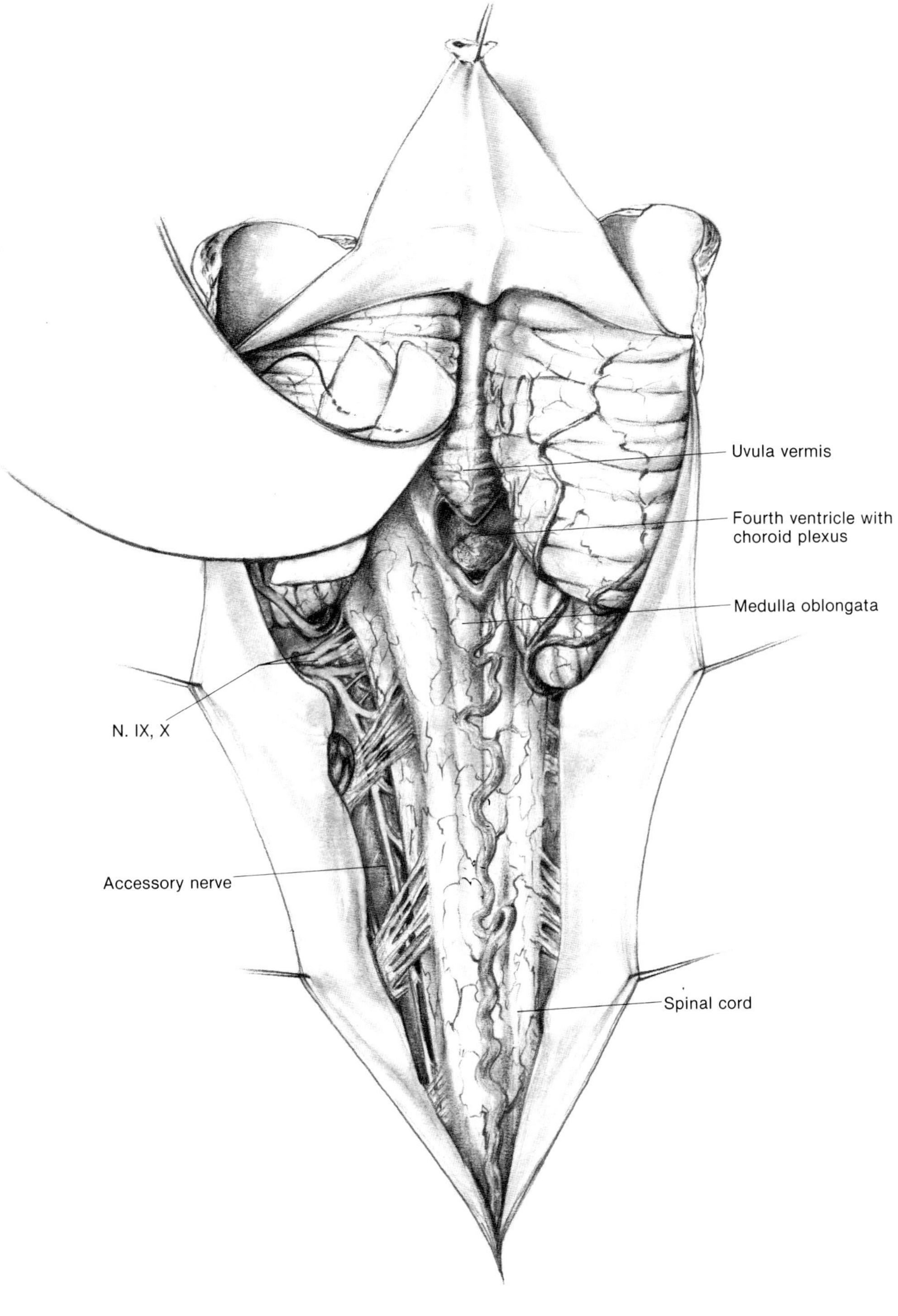

Fig. 10.4. View into the craniocervical junction and fourth ventricle following microsurgical tumor removal. The left cerebellar hemisphere, including the tonsil, is elevated with a spatula. The left caudal cranial nerves are visible

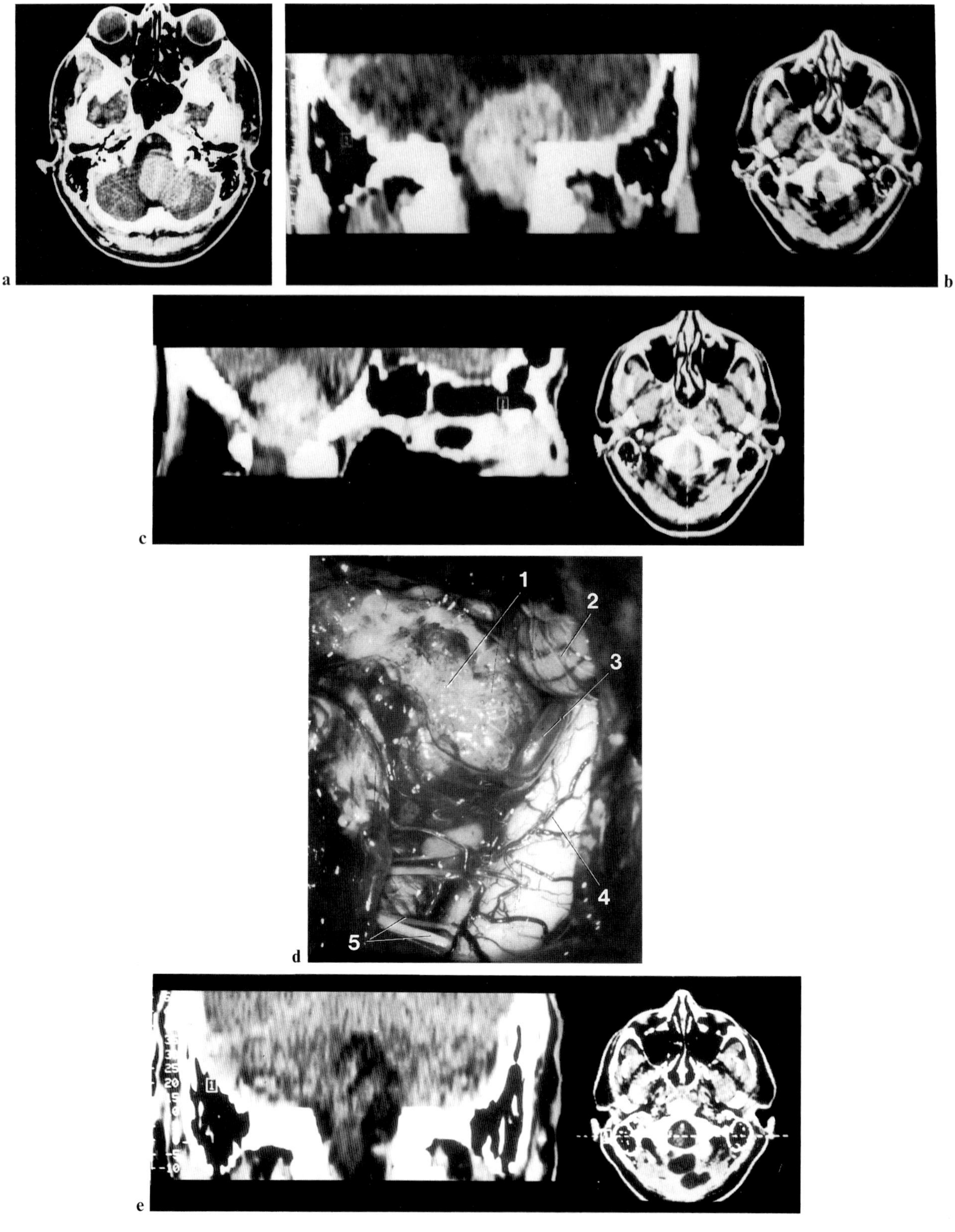
a
b
c
1
2
3
4
5
d
e

Illustrative Case

A 36-year-old man came to our attention because of a 2-year history of unsteady gait. Neurological examination disclosed decreased sensation on the right side and ataxic gait. CT scans showed a craniospinal meningioma (Fig. 10.5 a–c). Through a midline suboccipital craniectomy and after removal of the laminae of C1 and C2 a tumor located in correspondence of the anterior margin of the foramen magnum and pushing the craniocervical junction posterolaterally was completely removed (Fig. 10.5 d). The postoperative course was uncomplicated, and the patient was discharged, independent with an improved gait. Postoperative CT scans showed complete tumor removal (Fig. 10.5 e).

References

1. Cushing H, Eisenhardt C (1962) Meningiomas. Their classification, regional behavior, life history and surgical end results. Hafner, New York, pp 169–186
2. Kempe LG (1970) Operative neurosurgery, vol 2. Springer, Berlin Heidelberg New York, pp 45–53
3. Maxwell RE, Chou SN (1988) Posterior fossa meningiomas. In: Schmidek HH, Sweet WH (eds) Operative neurosurgical techniques: indications, methods and results, vol 1, 2nd edn. Grune and Stratton, New York, pp 571–582
4. Meyer FB, Ebersold MJ, Reese DF (1984) Benign tumors of the foramen magnum. J Neurosurg 61:136–142
5. Miller E, Crockard HA (1987) Transoral transclival removal of anteriorly located meningiomas at the foramen magnum. Neurosurgery 20:966–968
6. Ojemann RG (1985) Meningiomas: clinical features and surgical management. In: Wilkins RH, Rengachary SS (eds) Neurosurgery, vol 1. McGraw-Hill, New York, pp 648–651
7. Sen CN, Sekhar LN (1990) An extreme lateral approach to intradural lesions of the cervical spine and foramen magnum. Neurosurgery 27:197–204
8. Yasargil MG, Mortara RW, Curcic M (1980) Meningiomas of the basal posterior cranial fossa. In: Krayenbuhl H (ed) Advances and technical standards in neurosurgery, vol 7. Springer, Berlin Heidelberg New York, pp 3–115
9. Yasuoka S, Okazaki H, Daube JR, MacCarty CS (1978) Foramen magnum tumors. Analysis of 57 cases of benign extramedullary tumors. J Neurosurg 49:828–838

Fig. 10.5 a–e. Extensive meningioma at the left craniocervical junction in a 36-year-old man. The main clinical symptoms were hemihypoesthesia and hemihypalgesia, impaired termal sensation on the right side, and unsteady gait. **a** Axial CT scan covering the posterior fossa shows the large meningioma extending laterally into the cerebellopontine angle, anterior to the prepontine space, and posterior to the occiput. The tumor transgresses the midline. **b** Axial CT with coronal reconstruction to demonstrate the foramen magnum; half of the tumor is in the posterior fossa and half in the spinal canal. The foramen magnum is greatly constricted. **c** Axial CT scan with midsagittal reconstruction shows the relation of the tumor to the clivus, fourth ventricle, cisterna magna, and anterior arch of the atlas. **d** Status following suboccipital craniocervical exposure and elevation of the cerebellum and of the left tonsil. The tumor is displacing and compressing the brainstem and impinging on the upper cervical nerve roots and on the posterior inferior cerebellar artery. *1*, Tumor; *2*, cerebellar tonsil; *3*, posterior inferior cerebrellar artery; *4*, medulla oblongata; *5*, upper cervical nerve roots. **e** Postoperative CT scans

CHAPTER 11

Upper and Middle Clivus Meningiomas

General Considerations

Under the heading of upper and middle clivus meningiomas we include those operated upon when the tumor is located exclusively or mainly in correspondence of the upper and middle clivus. Only a few tumors fall into this group, and these represent the initial stage of tumors that with further growth would become petroclival, craniospinal, or incisural meningiomas. This view is supported by combined clinical and surgical observations showing that in many patients with petroclival, craniospinal, or incisural meningiomas the original symptoms were related to abducens paresis, often preceding by many years other symptoms and falsely diagnosed as strabism; moreover at surgery, in the same group of patients, many times the tumor attachment is found to be in proximity to the dural entrance or the intradural clival course of nerve VI, at the level of the middle-upper clivus. The reason why a counterpart does not exist in tumors originating from the lower clivus is the anatomical lack of a nervous structure which, like the abducens nerve, may be compressed by a still relatively small dural mass, resulting in a focal neurological deficit. The fact that these tumors are small at the time of surgery does not mean that their surgical removal is easier than that of larger meningiomas of this area (see "Surgical Considerations").

So defined, these tumors have not been previously described as a separate group but generally included with petroclival or incisural meningiomas.

Personal Series

Both of our two patients (Table 11.1) had been complaining of diplopia, at first intermittent, for a few years. Preoperatively both had abducens paresis and mild contralateral weakness, more marked in the arms. One patient, operated on at the beginning of this series, had a poor outcome due to postoperative intracerebellar bleeding. The other patient is independent and fully employable after the operation.

Surgical Considerations

Both tumors were nested in front of the brainstem at the level of the middle pons. Due to their relatively small size and the little mass effect, the neurovascular structures had not been significantly displaced by the tumor, and consequently the three surgical "corridors" that we usually employ to reach the clivus from a lateral suboccipital approach (below the nerve IX-XI complex, between the IX-XI and the VII-VIII complexes, and between the VII-VIII complex and nerve V) were very narrow, making tumor resection extremely difficult. A fourth surgical corridor, an artificial one created by large clival tumors bowing the tentorium superiorly between the trigeminal nerve and the undersurface

Table 11.1. Upper and middle clivus meningiomas

Number	2
Age: range/mean/median (years)	53 – 54/53.5/53.5
Women/men	2/0
Symptom (most common)	Double vision
Sign (most common)	Abducens paresis
Tumor removal	
Total	2
Subtotal	0
Outcome	
Good	1
Fair	0
Poor	1
Deaths	0

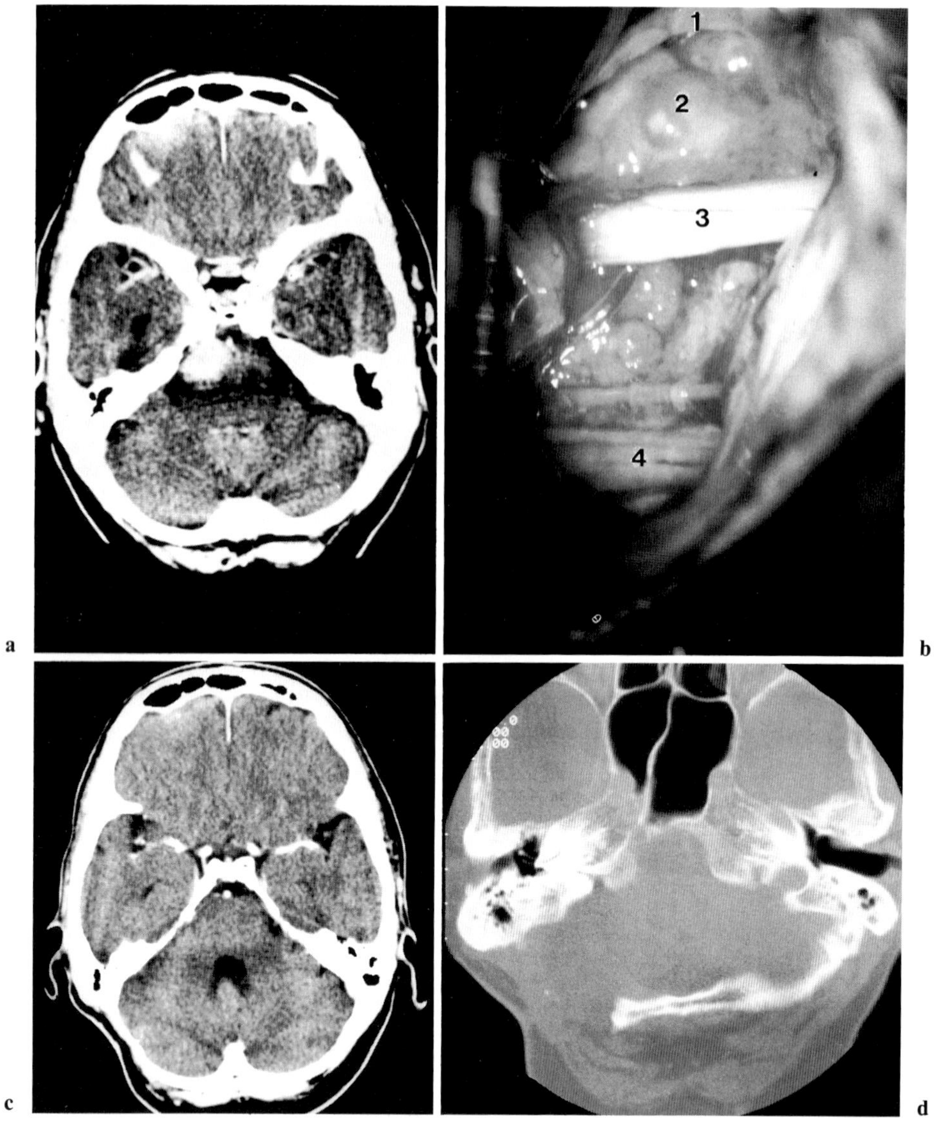

Fig. 11.1 a–d. Middle clival meningioma in a 63-year-old woman. **a** Preoperative CT scan shows the prepontine meningioma at the level of the middle clivus. **b** Intraoperative picture shows the mild posterior displacement of the nerve VII-VIII complex and the superior bowing of the trigeminal nerve. *1*, Trigeminal nerve; *2*, tumor; *3*, nerve VII-VIII complex; *4*, lower cranial nerves. **c, d** Postoperative CT scans show total tumor removal (**c**) and the craniotomy extent (**d**)

of the tent, is completely lacking in these medium-sized tumors. Consequently, in approaching these meningiomas through a lateral suboccipital craniectomy one must work at times in a very narrow area with the cerebellar vessels, especially the anterior inferior cerebellar artery, lying between the nerve VII-VIII complex and the tumor. Both cases were approached through a lateral suboccipital craniectomy medial to the sigmoid sinus. Having discussed the difficulties encountered in removing these tumors, we do not think that they would have been any less by using a combined supra-infratentorial presigmoid-sinus avenue or by using a subtemporal or a transsylvian approach. We do think that a transoral approach lends itself well anatomically to the treatment of this medium-sized middle-upper clival lesion, with the caveats related to the use of a transoral approach for the treatment of an intradural lesion.

Illustrative Case

A 63-year-old woman came to our attention with a 2-year history of double vision when looking to the right. Neurological examination disclosed a right abducens paresis and a left hemiparesis, worse in the arm. Audiogram showed a 50 dB hearing loss between 1.5 and 3 kH on the right. CT and MRI scans demonstrated a right prepontine extraxial mass at the level of the middle pons. The patient was operated on in the semisitting position with the head tilted 30° to the right and slightly flexed. A lateral suboccipital craniectomy was used to expose the right cerebellar hemisphere flush to the petrous pyramid. (For details of the surgical technique see Chap. 12.) The dura was opened just medial to the sigmoid sinus, and cerebrospinal fluid was drained from the lateral cerebellomedullary cistern. After medial retraction of the cerebellar hemisphere and visual exploration of the lower cerebellopontine cistern it was evident that the lower cranial nerves (IX–XI) as well as the VII-VIII complex were mildly displaced posteriorly by the prepontine mass. Nerve V was posterosuperiorly displaced. The tumor was completely removed working around the nerve VII-VIII complex. During tumor removal the auditory evoked potential were permanently lost, and nerve VIII was consequently cut, making tumor removal somewhat easier. The tumor originated from the dural entrance of nerve VI which was, both proximally and distally to this point, totally engulfed by tumor. It was possible to remove the tumor completely, preserving the nerve VI function. In addition to loss of the nerve VIII function, the postoperative neurological examination showed decreased hemiparesis and improvement of the abducens function, which returned to normal in 6 months (Fig. 11.1).

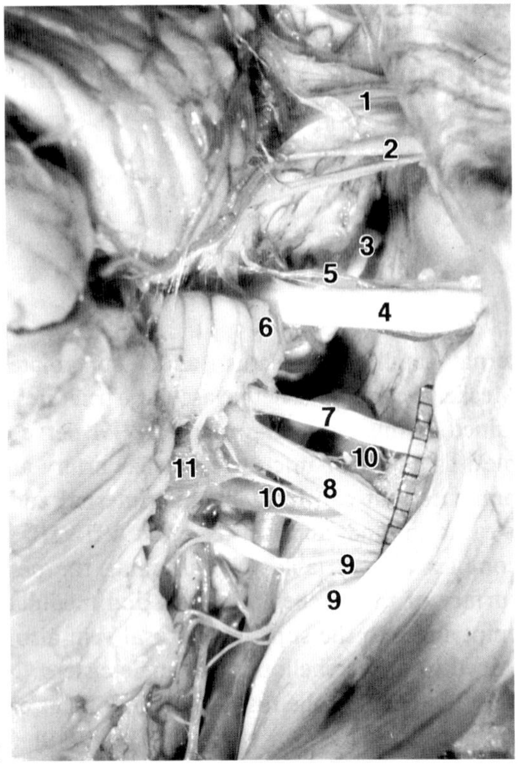

12.1

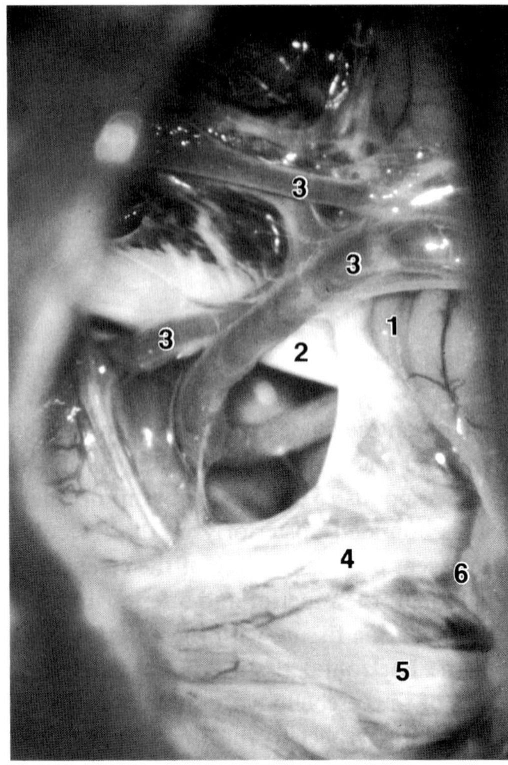

12.2

Fig. 12.1. The cerebellopontine angle and surrounding regions. *1*, Trigeminal nerve; *2*, petrosal vein; *3*, abducens nerve; *4*, VII-VIII nerve complex; *5*, anterior-inferior cerebellar artery; *6*, flocculus; *7*, *8*, *9*, cranial nerves IX, X, XI; *10*, posterior-inferior cerebellar artery; *11*, choroid plexus of the lateral recess of the fourth ventricle

Fig. 12.2. The arachnoid of the cerebellopontine angle cistern has been partially opened. The flocculus (*1*), the VII-VIII nerve complex (*2*), the anterior-inferior cerebellar artery and its branches (*3*) are well visualized. Cranial nerves IX (*4*) and X (*5*) are still covered by the arachnoid of the lateral cerebellar medullary cistern; the choroid plexus of the lateral recess of the fourth ventricle (*6*) is also evident

et al. [15] have reported different microsurgical series over the past 10 years. The term cerebellopontine angle meningioma, although widely used, is somewhat imprecise because, if it refers to the dural site of attachment, many of these tumors originate outside the cerebellopontine angle, and if it refers to the topographical encroachment of the tumor upon the cerebellopontine angle (differently from what happens with acoustic neurinomas, which originate within the angle), it brings together different surgical and clinical entities, such as those tumors originating anteriorly and posteriorly to the internal auditory meatus. The term meningioma of the posterior surface of the petrous pyramid, if used to denote the site of dural attachment would tend to exclude those meningiomas not originating from the posterior pyramid but growing in close relation to it, such as meningiomas of the undersurface of the tentorium and meningiomas of the lateral clivus. Moreover, at times even under the operating microscope the site of dural attachment may not be clear, or it may extend from one area to the other. For this reason, we prefer to use the term posterior pyramid meningiomas to topographically denote those tumors whose main direction of growth brings their major bulk in contact with the posterior pyramid, irrespective of their site of dural attachment. In addition, as the clinical presentation and the surgical problems differ depending on the relationship between the main tumor mass and the internal auditory meatus, respectively, anterior and posterior to it, we subdivide these tumors into those located anterior and those located posterior to the internal auditory meatus. Both elements of this proposed classification may be easily obtained by using CT scans (Fig. 12.6).

12.3 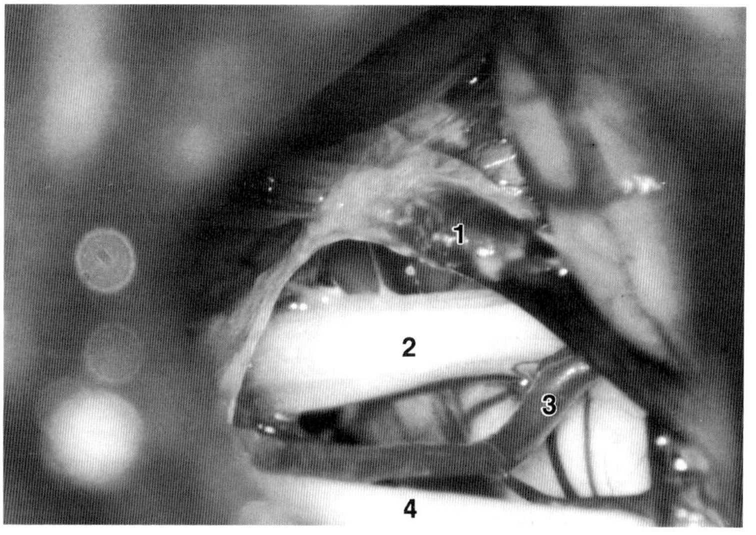

12.4 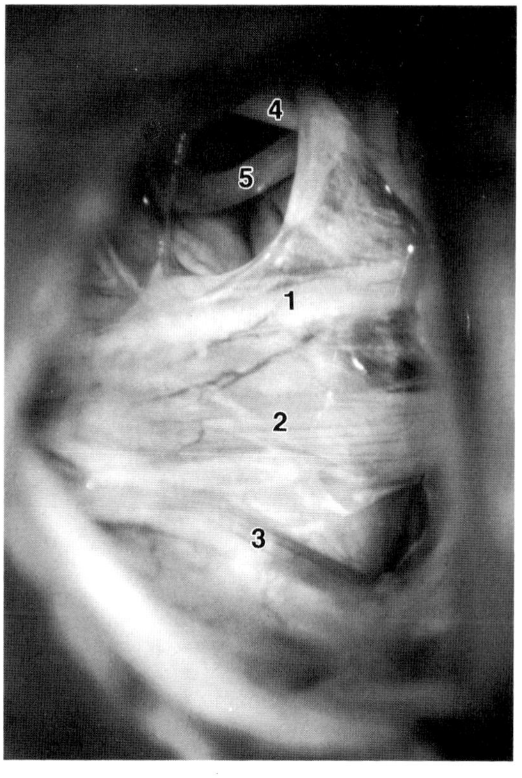

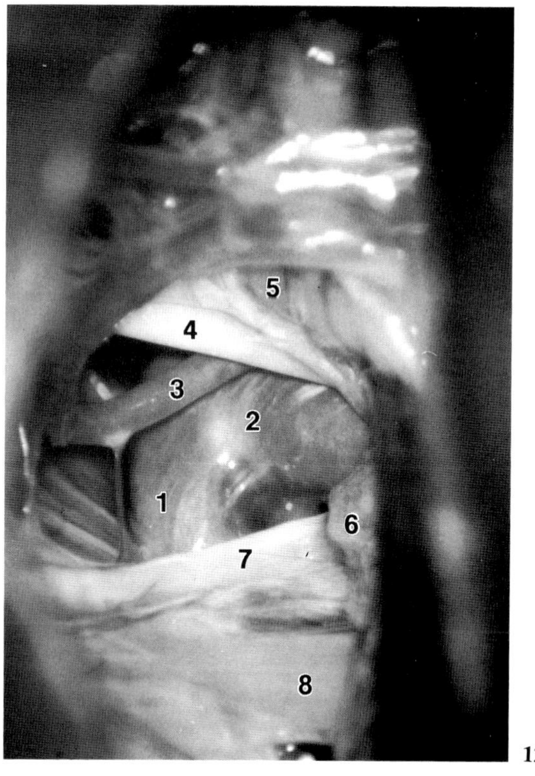 12.5

Fig. 12.3. The rostral portion of the cerebellopontine angle cistern contains the petrosal vein (*1*) and the trigeminal nerve (*2*), usually enveloped by thickened arachnoid. Anterior/inferior cerebellar artery branches (*3*) are visualized. The lower portion of the illustration shows the VII-VIII nerve complex (*4*)

Fig. 12.4. The arachnoid of the lower part of the cerebellopontine angle cistern has been opened to demonstrate the relationship between this cistern and the lateral cerebellomedullary cistern. Through the intact arachnoid of the lateral cerebellomedullary cistern one can see cranial nerves IX (*1*), X (*2*), and XI (*3*). The lower portion of the VII-VIII nerve complex (*4*) and a loop of the anterior-inferior cerebellar artery (*5*) are also visible

Fig. 12.5. The arachnoid at the junction of the lateral cerebellomedullary cistern with the cerebellopontine angle cistern has been opened. The vertebral artery (*1*), the origin of the posterior-inferior cerebellar artery (*2*), a loop of the anterior-inferior cerebellar artery (*3*), and the lower portion of the VII-VIII nerve complex (*4*) are well seen. The flocculus (*5*), the choroid plexus of the lateral recess of the fourth ventricle (*6*), and cranial nerves IX (*7*) and X (*8*) are also identifiable

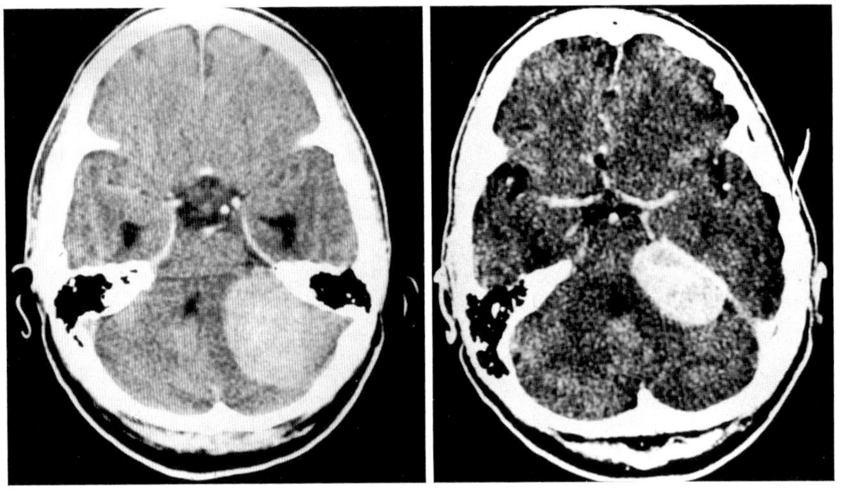

Fig. 12.6 a, b. CT scans of meningiomas of the posterior pyramid. **a** One located posterior to the internal auditory meatus. **b** One located anterior to the internal auditory meatus

Personal Series

Our material is presented in Table 12.1. It can be seen that there is a difference in clinical presentation between the tumors located posteriorly and anteriorly to the internal auditory meatus, the former presenting with cerebellar symptoms and signs and the latter with decreased hearing. The mean and median tumor size were the same in the two groups (4 cm), with a wider range in the anterior group (2.5–6 vs 3–5 cm). The interval between the onset of symptoms and the diagnosis was quite different in the two groups, with a median interval of 1 year (mean 10 months, range 2 weeks to 2 years) in the posterior group and a median interval of 3 years (mean 4.3 years, range 5 weeks to 15 years) in the anterior group.

The differences between the two groups are also highlighted when one looks at the tumor extension into the surrounding areas: the tumor extended to the lower clivus in one patient, to and above the incisura in two, and to the foramen magnum and incisura in one among the posterior group, while among the tumors located anterior to the internal auditory meatus the foramen magnum, incisura, and clivus were involved in seven cases, the foramen magnum and incisura in one, and the incisura in six. An en plaque component was found three times in the anterior group and never in the posterior. In the anterior group there was one case of a tumor growing inside ventricle IV through the lateral recess (Fig. 12.7). In the posterior group the tumor attachment was at the level of the tentorium in eight cases, at the jugular foramen in one, and on the petrous pyramid immediately posterior to the internal auditory meatus in three. In the anterior group, the tumor attachment was on the petrous pyramid immediately anterior to the internal auditory meatus in ten patients, on other areas of the

Fig. 12.7 a–d. Meningioma of the right cerebellopontine angle and fourth ventricle. **a** Mass lesion of the right posterior cranial fossa 4 cm in diameter extending across the midline from the posterior surface of the petrous pyramid and completely filling the fourth ventricle. **b** The tumor is exposed in the cerebellopontine angle between the trigeminal nerve above and the vestibulocochlear and facial nerves below. *1*, Spatula; *2*, trigeminal nerve; *3*, tumor; *4*, cranial nerves VII and VIII. **c** The cerebellopontine angle has been cleared of tumor, permitting identification of cranial nerves VII and VIII, the anterior inferior cerebellar artery and the caudal cranial nerve group. *1*, Cranial nerves VII and VIII; *2*, caudal cranial nerves; *3*, anterior inferior cerebellar artery; *4*, brain spatula. **d** The intraventricular tumor component has been removed from the fourth ventricle. This picture shows a view from the right lateral aspect through the enlarged foramen of Luschka onto the floor and opposite lateral wall of the fourth ventricle. *1*, Floor of fourth ventricle; *2*, loop of posterior inferior cerebellar artery; *3*, cerebral aqueduct; *4*, cerebellum

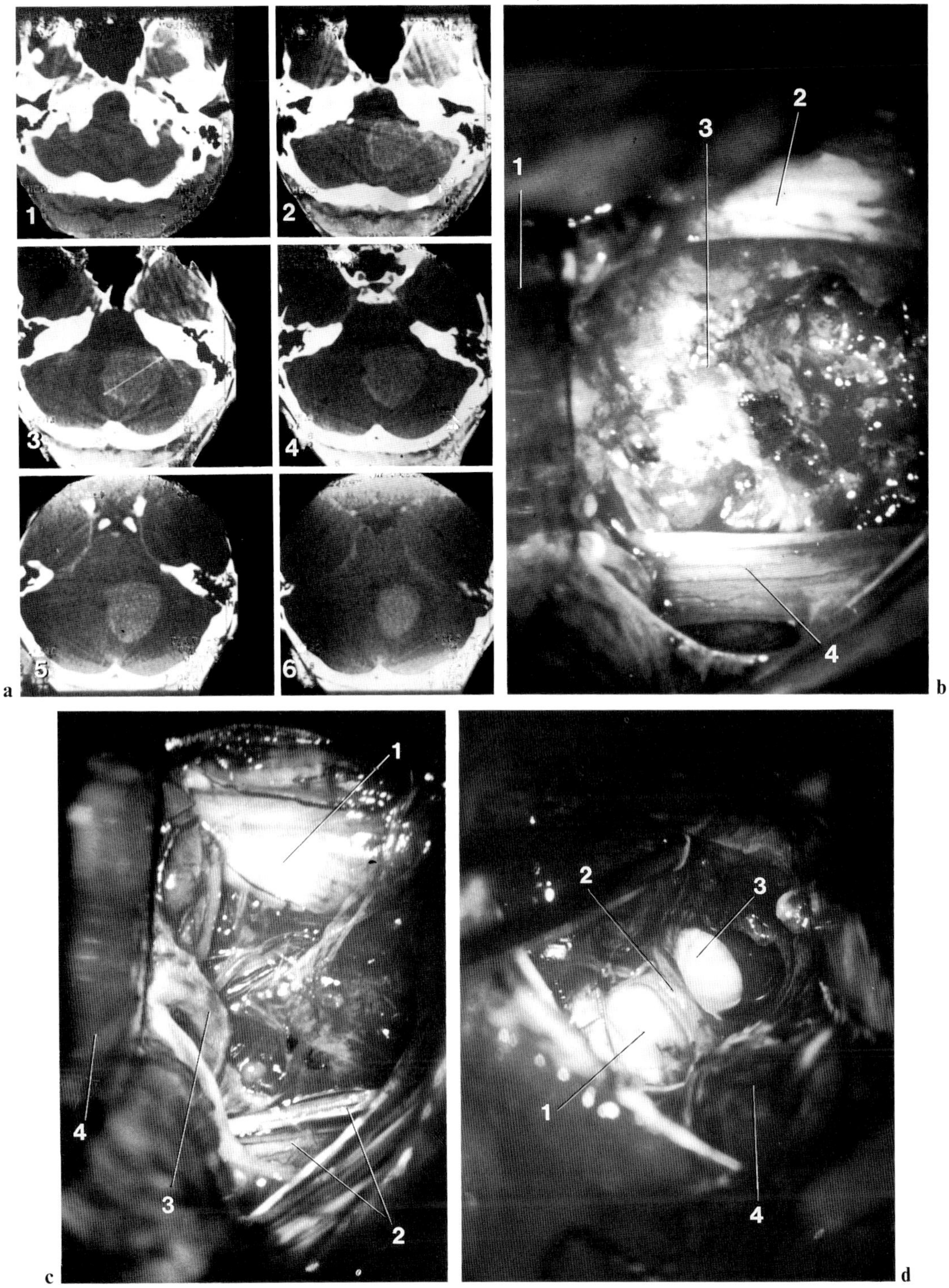
a
b
c
d

Table 12.1. Posterior pyramid meningiomas

Tumors located anterior to the internal auditory meatus	
Number	32
Age: range/mean/median (years)	33 – 76/53/52.5
Women/men	24/8
Symptom (most common)	Abnormal hearing
Sign (most common)	Decreased nerve VIII function
Tumor removal	
Total	29
Subtotal	3
Outcome	
Good	28
Fair	3
Poor	1
Deaths	0
Tumors located posterior to the internal auditory meatus	
Number	24
Age: range/mean/median (years)	23 – 72/57/55
Women/men	21/3
Symptom (most common)	Trouble walking
Sign (most common)	Cerebellar signs
Tumor removal	
Total	24
Subtotal	0
Outcome	
Good	22
Fair	2
Poor	0
Deaths	0

petrous pyramid anterior to the internal auditory meatus in six, on the tentorium in ten, between the internal auditory meatus and the jugular foramen in three, and diffuse en plaque in the region of the clivus in three. Hydrocephalus requiring shunting was present twice in the anterior group and once in the posterior group. In the anterior group, due to tumor invasion, nerves V and VI had to be cut once, nerve VII had to be sacrificed three times, and nerve VIII twice. In the posterior group, cranial nerve morbidity was significantly lower; we had to sacrifice only once nerve VIII. There was one patient in the anterior group whose en plaque tumor progressed with brainstem compression despite subtotal tumor removal and radiation therapy. He underwent a "total" tumor removal with sacrifice of nerves IV–VIII. Of the 32 patients with anteriorly located tumors, 28 are independent, 3 need some degree of assistance, and one patient operated in a comatose status needs continuous assistance. Of the 24 patients with posteriorly located tumors, 22 are independent, and two need occasional assistance. We believe that the differences in clinical presentation and the surgical differences are a direct consequence of the different anatomical location, with the anteriorly placed tumors having larger cisterns to accommodate their expansion.

Surgical Consideration

In the microneurosurgical era, these tumors have been approached mainly through a lateral suboccipital craniectomy or craniotomy, with the patient in the semisitting or three-quarters prone supine position [12, 17, 20]. We operate on these tumors with the patient in the semisitting position, the head secured in a three-point Mayfield frame, flexed and turned 30° toward the side of the lesion. By moving the whole head foreward, it is possible even in patients with a short neck to flex the head adequately without comprimising the cephalic venous return. This is checked by leaving enough space to accommodate two fingers between the patient's chin and sternum. The aim of the position is to place the posteroanterior axis of the petrous pyramid in a line corresponding to the surgeon's line of vision. The patient's knees and hips are mildly flexed while the upper trunk leans backward about 20° from the vertical plane. The patient's legs are fitted with elastic stockings; a precordial Doppler, end-tidal CO_2, and a central line catheter are routine means for early detection and treatment of air emboli. A vertical 10-cm skin incision is made about one finger's breath medial to the posterior margin of the mastoid, extending from approximately 2 cm above the superior nuchal line (Fig. 12.8a). A routine subperiosteal exposure of the occipital squama and the medial aspect of the mastoid is executed. A suboccipital craniectomy is then performed, placing one burrhole over the expected confluence of the transverse and sigmoid sinus, that is, usually around the junction of the superior nuchal line with the base of the mastoid.

A circular craniectomy about 3 – 3.5 cm in diameter is then performed. The craniectomy should expose the inferior border of the transverse sinus superiorly, the angle between the transverse and sigmoid sinus, and the medial edge of the sigmoid sinus laterally and should extend as low as neces-

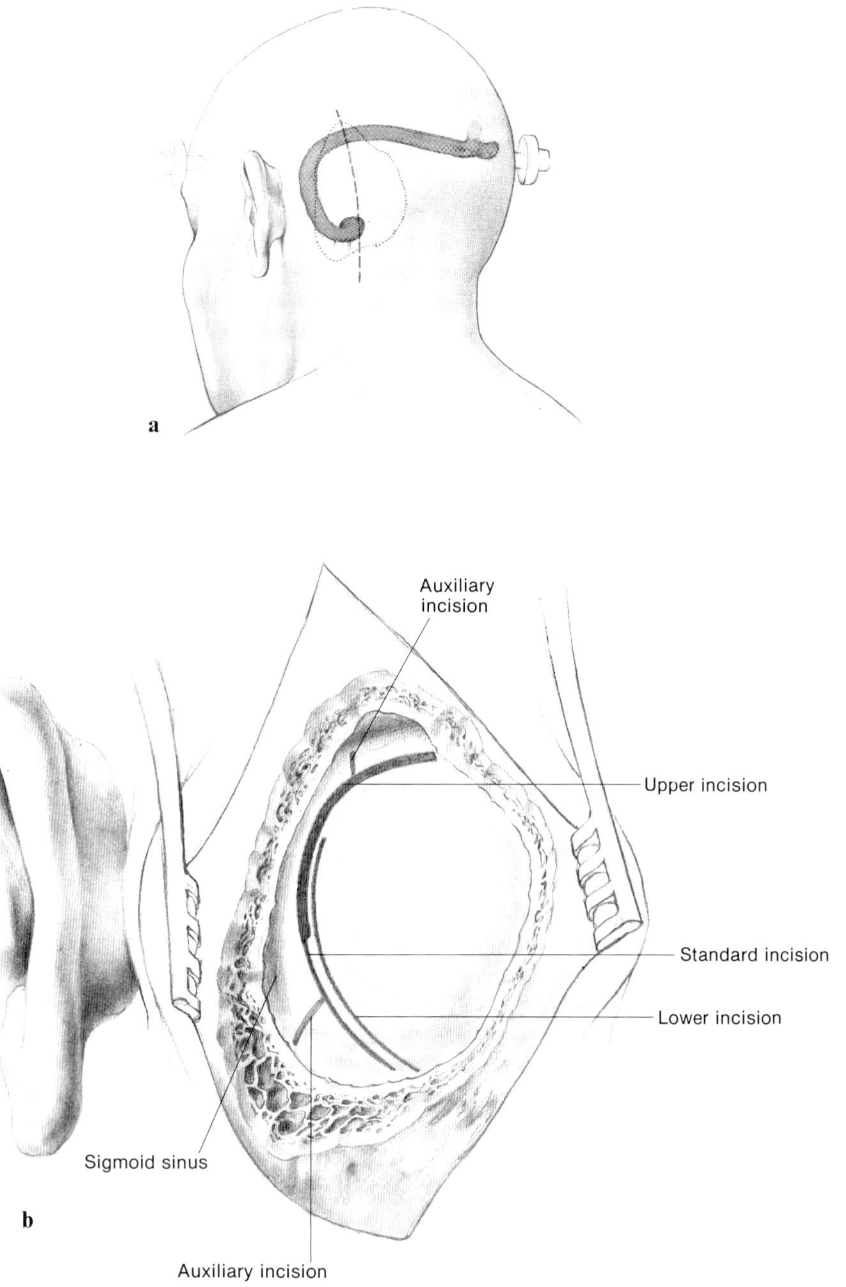

Fig. 12.8 a, b. The lateral suboccipital (retrosigmoid) approach to the internal auditory canal and cerebellopontine angle. **a** A vertical skin incision approximately 10 cm long is placed 1.5–2 cm medial to the mastoid. It extends superiorly to the level of the transverse sinus. Its inferior extent depends on whether the lesion is at the level of the superior or inferior cranial nerves. **b** After retraction of the soft tissues and muscles, a burrhole is placed below the junction of the transverse and sigmoid sinuses and enlarged to 2–3 cm with a rongeur. The sigmoid sinus must be exposed regardless of the extent of mastoid pneumatization. This improves vision of the cerebellopontine angle and minimizes retraction of the cerebellum. The possible dural incisions are indicated and depend on the surgical goal. The "standard incision" is for exposing the entire cerebellopontine angle from the tentorial incisure to the foramen magnum. The upper incision is for exposing the trigeminal nerve, the lower incision for exposing cranial nerves VII and VIII and the caudal nerve group. The "auxiliary" incisions create dural flaps that are retracted with holding sutures to improve access

sary to fully expose the horizontal portion of the occipital squama (Fig. 12.8b). If the tumor extends low into the posterior fossa around the jugular foramen, the bottom of the craniectomy is lowered accordingly, reaching toward but not to the foramen magnum. The bone over the sinus may be removed using a high-speed drill after careful dural separation. A few diploic or emissary veins draining into the sinus may be encountered. These are coagulated away from the sinus and then sharply transsected. If a hole or small tear is made in the sinus, it is usually packed with Gelfoam, held in place by a cottonoid. Bigger tears need to be sutured. Opened mastoid cells may be sealed with bone wax. From this time on, until the dura is closed, the operation is performed using the operating microscope. The dura is cut in a C-shape 3 to 4 mm medial to the sigmoid sinus flush with the transverse sinus, extending well over the horizontal portion of the occipital squama (Fig. 12.8b). The lateral edge of the dura is then put under tension using 4-0 sutures attached to hemostats. The lateral cerebellomedullary cistern is then opened under direct vision, and cerebrospinal fluid is allowed to escape, relaxing the cerebellum. If there is no cerebrospinal fluid to let out because the cistern is filled with tumor, one may decide immediately to debulk the tumor, or to open the cisterna magna, or to tap the occipital horn. At this stage the cerebellum, exposed only on its lateral 1.0–1.5 cm, is covered with cottonoid and gently retracted posteromedially. The tumor is usually evident at this time; its posterior capsule, which is nothing but thickened arachnoid, is opened, and the relationship of the tumor to the cranial nerves is assessed.

In the posterior group the VII-VIII nerve complex was generally pushed anteriorly, but in one case it was pushed cranially and in one caudally (Fig. 12.9). In the anterior group the VII-VIII nerve complex was displaced posteriorly or caudally with equal frequency, and in only three cases was it displaced cranially (Fig. 12.10). Nerve V was usually displaced cranially, but it was displaced caudally twice and posteriorly once. The lower cranial nerves (IX-XI) were always displaced inferiorly other than in one instance in which they were displaced posteriorly. Once the tumor is exposed, it is removed by alternating intratumoral decompression using the ultrasonic aspiration, the laser, or the bipolar microforceps-microscissors with extracapsular separation of the tumor from the surrounding neurovascular structures. While there is usually a good cleavage arachnoidal plane between the tumor and vessels, nerve and brain, we have found in quite a few instances the tumor completely surrounding but not invading nerves and vessels. In this situation, the only way to preserve function is

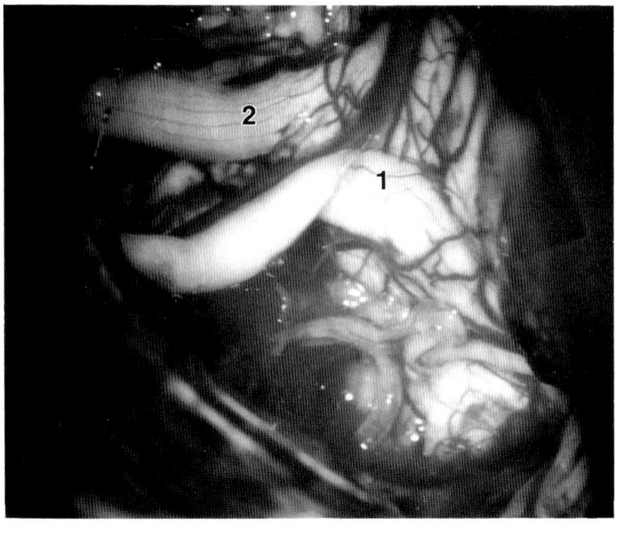

Fig. 12.9. The anterosuperior bowing of the VII-VIII nerve complex is evident at the end of the removal of a posteriorly located meningioma. *1*, VII-VIII nerve complex; *2*, trigeminal nerve

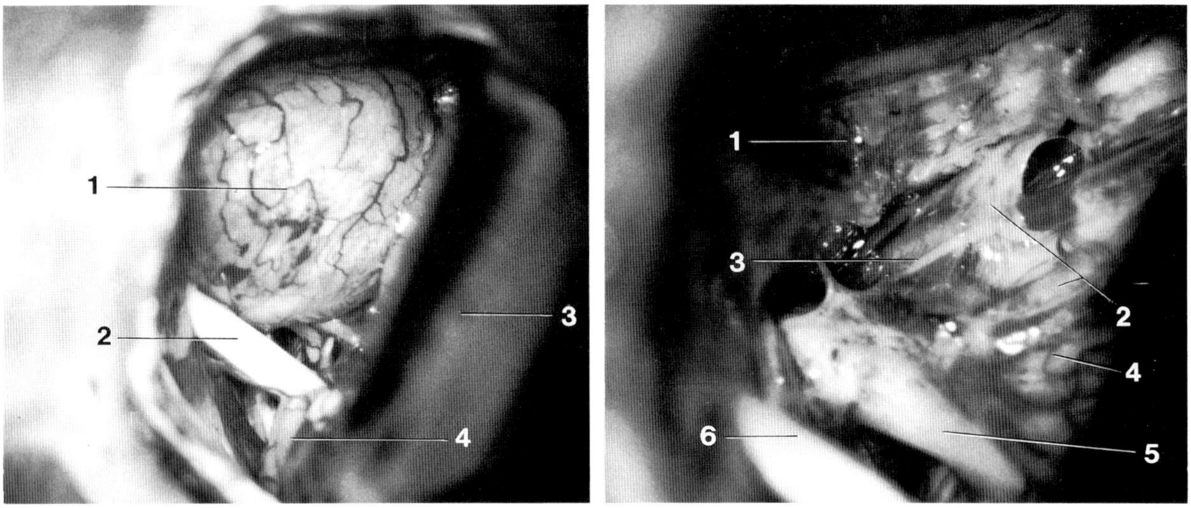

Fig. 12.10 a, b. Meningioma of the posterior pyramid located anterior to the internal auditory meatus and originating from the undersurface of the tentorium. **a** Status following lateral suboccipital exposure of the cerebellopontine angle. The smooth, globular tumor occupies the space between the tentorium above, the brainstem medially, nerves VII and VIII below, and the posterior surface of the pyramid. The trigeminal nerve and trochlear nerve are covered by the tumor. *1*, Tumor; *2*, cranial nerves VII and VIII; *3*, brain spatula; *4*, flocculus. **b** Status following tumor removal. The tentorial attachment of the tumor is coagulated before the tumor is removed. The major neurovascular structures of the cerebellopontine angle are exposed. *1*, Tumor attachment on tentorium; *2*, branches of superior cerebellar artery; *3*, trochlear nerve; *4*, brainstem; *5*, trigeminal nerve; *6*, cranial nerves VII and VIII

carefully to dissect the tumor away from the neurovascular structures starting at a place where these two structures are already separated. In an en plaque tumor, it is usually not possible to develop this plane, and at times, even in tumors that have an expansive type of growth, we have found definite evidence of infiltration of nerves.

In the process of tumor removal, an attempt should be made to interrupt the main vascular pedicle of the tumor that often comes from the petrous bone. If this is done, the tumor softens, and its removal becomes easier and entails less blood loss. These tumors may at times grow with little finger-like expansions toward the brainstem, indenting it very deeply, and great care must be paid in removing these tumor extensions. Occasionally we have found it useful for reaching the superior pole of the tumor to develop a corridor between the undersurface of the tent and the trigeminal nerve. Generally, the VII-VIII nerve complex is well defined, and especially the facial nerve is more easily recognizable in these tumors than in acoustic tumors, where this nerve is elongated and its bulk sometimes longitudinally split.

At the end of tumor resection, attention is given to eliminate the dural site of attachment and to drill off any abnormal area of bone. We needed to drill the internal auditory meatus nine times in the anterior group and twice in the posterior group. The jugular foramen was drilled twice in the anterior group and once in the posterior group. The opened internal auditory meatus is closed with a small piece of muscle fixed with fibrin glue. Hemostasis is then secured and double-checked with a Valsalva maneuver that sometimes reveals venous bleeding not evident before. The dura is closed in a water-tight fashion with a continuous suture, and the muscles and skin are closed as usual. A compressive dressing is then applied for about 1 week.

Illustrative Cases

Tumors Located Anterior to the Internal Auditory Meatus. A 55-year-old man presented to us with left-sided deafness of 1-year duration. Neurological examination, other than for the left ear deafness was unremarkable. CT scan showed an homogeneously enhancing tumor of the left posterior pyra-

12.11 a

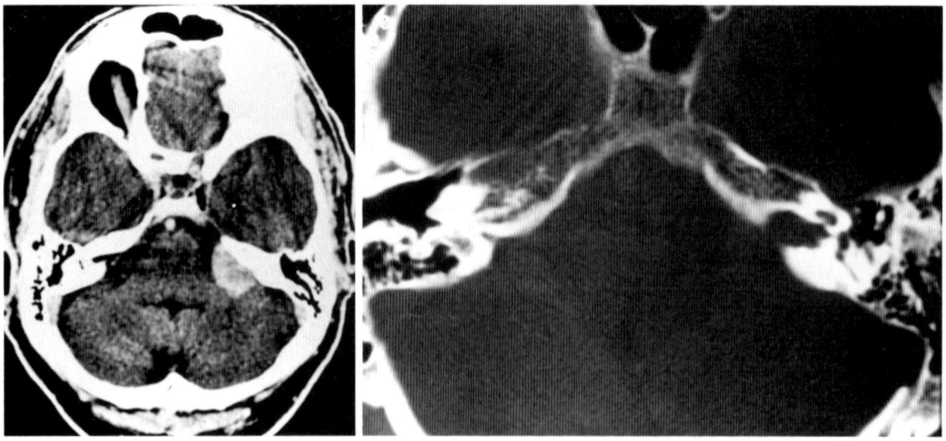

b

12.12 a

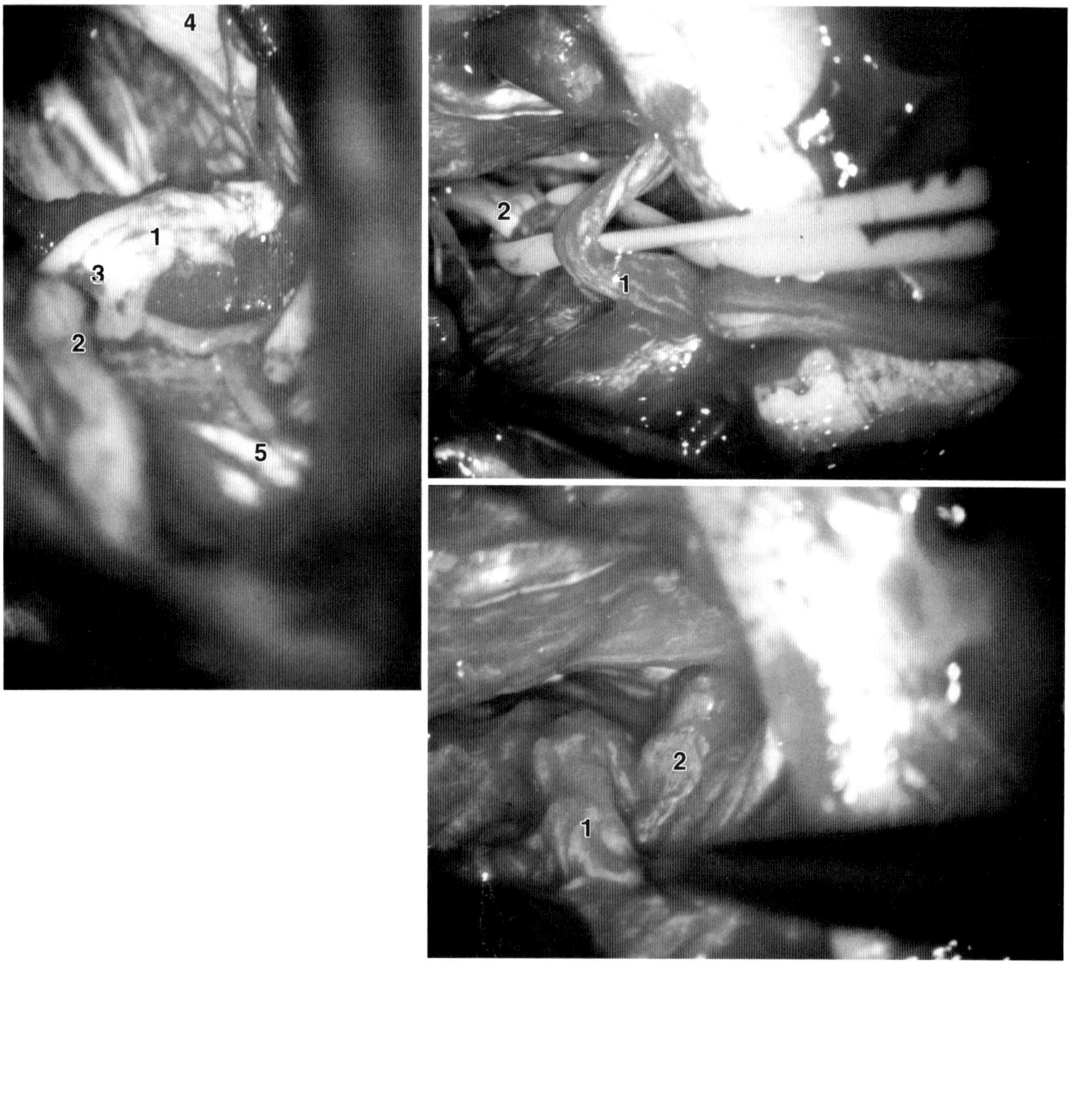

b

c

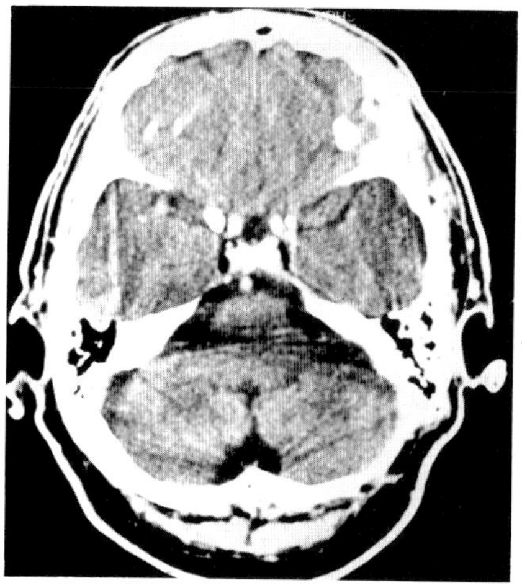

12.13

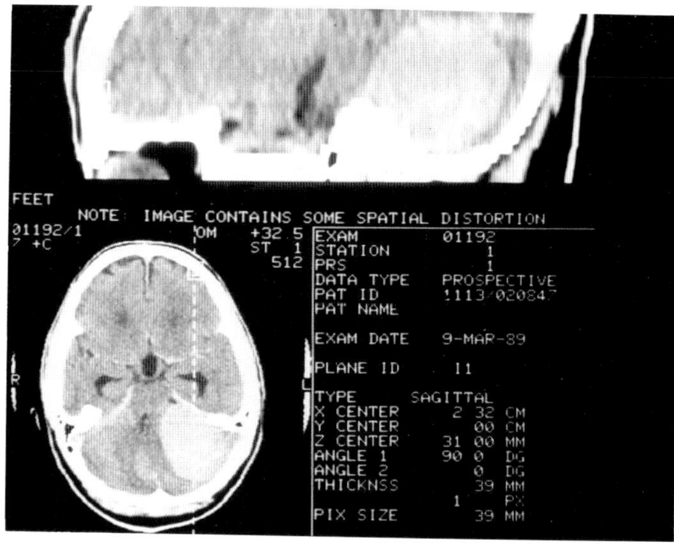

12.14

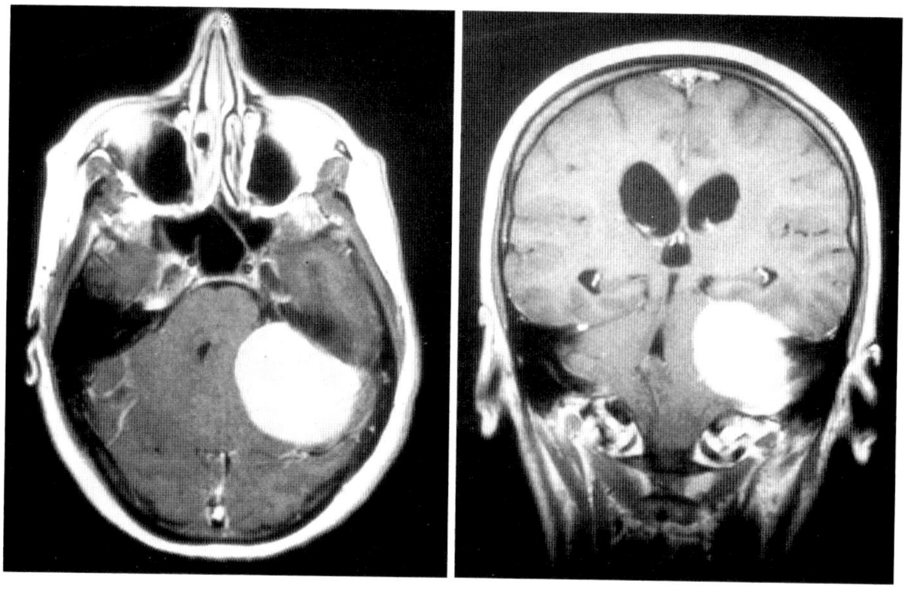

12.15a b

Fig. 12.11. **a.** CT scan of a left cerebellopontine angle meningioma located anterior to the internal auditory meatus. **b** The enlargement of the internal auditory meatus is well imaged using the bony technique

Fig. 12.12a–c. One-stage intracranial-extracranial anastomosis of the facial nerve following removal of a cerebellopontine angle meningioma involving the facial nerve. **a** The central stump of the facial nerve has been anastomized in the cerebellopontine angle to the sural nerve graft using fibrin glue. *1*, Central facial nerve stump; *2*, sural nerve graft; *3*, anastomosis; *4*, trigeminal nerve; *5*, caudal cranial nerves. **b** The sural nerve graft has been brought extracranially next to the peripheral facial nerve isolated near the stylomastoid foramen. *1*, Sural nerve graft; *2*, peripheral facial nerve. **c** The anastomosis has been completed. *1*, Sural nerve graft; *2*, peripheral facial nerve

Fig. 12.13. Postoperative CT scan showing total removal of a cerebellopontine angle meningioma originating anterior to the internal auditory meatus

Fig. 12.14. CT scan, axial cut and sagittal reconstruction of a posterior pyramid (cerebellopontine angle) meningioma located posterior to the internal auditory meatus. The shift of ventricle IV and the obstructive noncommunicating hydrocephalus are well imaged

Fig. 12.15a, b. Gadolinium-enhanced MRI shows an intensely enhancing lesion in the left posterior pyramid. The shift of the ventricle IV and of the brainstem as well as the ventricular enlargement are well imaged. **a** Axial view. **b** Coronal view

3. De Martel T, Guillaume J (1934) Méningiome du trou auditif interne. Ablation. Guérison. Rev Neurol (Paris) 62:66–68
4. De Martel T, Thurel R (1936) Méningiome de la region de l'angle pontocérébelleux. Rev Oto Neuro Ophtalmol (Paris) 14:110–112
5. Grand W, Bakay L (1975) Posterior fossa meningiomas. A report of 30 cases. Acta Neurochir (Wien) 32: 219–233
6. Henschen F (1910) Über Geschwulste der hinteren Schädelgrube, insbesondere des Kleinhirnbrückenwinkels. Fischer, Jena
7. Henschen F (1912) Die Acusticustumoren, eine neue Gruppe radiographisch darstellbarer Hirntumoren. RO-FO 18:207–216
8. Hoffman GR, de Busscher J, de Haene A (1957) Le méningiome de l'angle pontocerebelleux. Neurochirurgia (Stuttg) 3:123–137
9. Markham JW, Fager CA, Horrax G et al. (1955) Meningiomas of the posterior fossa. Their diagnosis, clinical features and surgical treatment. Arch Neurol Psychiatry 74:163–170
10. Matsumo H, Rhoton AL, Peace D (1982) Microsurgical anatomy of the posterior fossa cisterns. Neurosurgery 23:58–80
11. Matsushima T, Rhoton AL, Lenkey C (1982) Neurosurgery of the fourth ventricle. I. Neurosurgery 11: 631
12. Ojemann RG (1985) Meningiomas: clinical features and surgical management. In: Wilkins RH, Rengachary SS (eds) Neurosurgery, vol 1. McGraw-Hill, New York, pp 648–651
13. Petit-Dutalis D, Daum S (1949) Les méningiomes de la fosse postérieure. Rev Neurol 81:557–572
14. Russell JR, Bucy PC (1953) Meningiomas of the posterior fossa. Surg Gynecol Obstet 96:183–192
15. Samii M, Turel KE, Penkert G (1985) Management of seventh and eighth nerve involvement by cerebellopontine angle tumors. Clin Neurosurg 32:242–272
16. Scott M (1972) The surgical management of the meningiomas of the posterior fossa. Surg Gynecol Obstet 135:545–550
17. Sekhar LN, Jannetta PJ (1984) Cerebellopontine angle meningiomas. Microsurgical excision and follow-up results. J Neurosurg 60:500–505
18. Virchow R (1863–1865) Die krankhaften Geschwulste. Dreißig Vorlesungen, gehalten während des Wintersemesters 1862–1863 an der Universität zu Berlin, 2 vols. Hirschwald, Berlin
19. Yasargil MG (1984) Microneurosurgery, vol 1. Thieme, Stuttgart, pp 47–52
20. Yasargil MG, Mortara RW, Curcic M (1980) Meningiomas of the basal posterior cranial fossa. In: Krayenbühl H (ed) Advances and technical standards in neurosurgery, vol 7. Springer, Berlin Heidelberg New York, pp 3–115

CHAPTER 13

Petroclival Meningiomas

General Considerations

The present system of classification of petroclival meningiomas and of posterior fossa meningiomas in general is largely inadequate. The amount of information that it conveys is at times confused, misleading, and insufficient to allow for meaningful comparisons of different series. This problem is discussed in Chap. 12, and it is of even more relevance in the context of petroclival meningiomas. If a petroclival meningioma is one involving the apical petrous bone and the clivus without further qualification, many of our meningiomas of the anterior group of the posterior pyramid should be labeled as petroclival meningiomas, but this is inappropriate because the main direction of growth and the main bulk of these tumors are more posterior, and their surgical problems are different from those of petroclival meningiomas. On the other hand, if the dural attachment, sometimes diffuse and not always precisely identifiable [12], is the determining criterion, small meningiomas of the clivus, apical petrous bone, or petroclival synchondrosis should be considered petroclival meningiomas, although their surgical problems, outcome, etc. are different from those of larger tumors – while meningiomas arising from the tentorial notch but whose direction of growth leads them to extend well below the incisura to involve the petrous bone and clivus should not be considered petroclival meningiomas.

Considering today's capabilities for aggressive removal of these tumors, what is most important therefore is the topographical location of the main tumor bulk as it relates to the bony skull base. We stress here, as we have in other chapters, the relationship between the tumor and the skull base, because it is the bony skull base that is between the tumor and the outside world; it is the skull base that needs to be removed to attack the tumor, and it is the relationship between the bony skull base and the main tumor bulk that dictates the surgical approach. A system that assesses these relationships objectively using neuroradiological means would probably contribute greatly to the solution of this nosological problem; this is not a theoretical but a practical concern and involves further standardization and consequently more rational treatment. In the absence of such a system we are forced to rely on rather elusive terms, and we prefer, in this case as in others, to use a topographical term that takes into account the main tumor bulk and its direction of growth. Consequently we mean by petroclival meningioma a tumor whose main bulk is located over the petrous apex and the upper clivus; these tumors are usually large (> 25 cm) and usually extend through the incisura in the supratentorial compartment and for a variable length over the middle clivus.

Before 1970 the surgical mortality associated with the removal of meningiomas originating from the petrous apex and clivus was over 50%, and total resection was reported in only one of the 26 cases operated on to that date [8]. Consequently, it was not surprising that Castellano and Ruggiero [2], when reviewing Olivecrona's series considered clival meningiomas inoperable. Since the introduction and refinement of microneurosurgical techniques and approaches there have been a few reports of series with a mortality rate under 10% [8, 12] and a few with 0% mortality [1, 10].

Personal Series

The most important data of our series are summarized in Table 13.1. The average interval between the onset of symptoms and the diagnosis was 2.5 years, but there was one patient who started to

Table 13.1. Petroclival meningiomas

Number	27
Age: range/mean/median (years)	25 – 64/45/42
Women/men	20/7
Symptom (most common)	Unsteady gait
Sign (most common)	Decreased nerve VIII function
Tumor removal	
Total	20
Subtotal	7
Outcome	
Good	20
Fair	3
Poor	4
Deaths	0

complain of trigeminal neuralgia on the side of the tumor 16 years before the diagnosis was made. In our series 67% (18/27) of tumors were larger than 2.5 cm in major diameter, with many being 5 cm or more. The tumor extended above the tentorial notch in 41% (11/27) of cases and was at or below the foramen magnum 18% (5/27) of the times. The most common presenting symptom was unsteady gait, usually a combination of cerebellar gait and mild weakness reflecting brainstem compression, and the most common sign was decreased hearing. Total tumor removal was achieved in 74% (20/27) of cases. The most common postoperative problem was cranial nerve deficit involving principally the facial and cochlear nerve. Three patients had persistent facial palsy treated with a XII-VII anastomosis (two cases) or a facio-facial anastomosis (one case). Trochlear nerve palsy was present in six and abducens palsy in one patient. Hemiparesis was seen in three cases and temporary aphasia in two. After the operation 74% (20/27) of our patients were fully independent.

Surgical Considerations

The proximity of the petroclival region to the brainstem, to the vertebrobasilar arterial system, and to cranial nerve III-XII makes its surgical exposure extremely difficult. In addition, tumors located in this area usually attain a considerable size before the diagnosis is made, and consequently the relationships between the tumor and the surrounding neurovascular structures are extremely complex, with the cranial nerves and arteries often being engulfed by the tumor. Limited exposure of this area may be achieved through a frontotemporal craniotomy incising the tentorium and drilling off the petrous apex, through a posterior subtemporal craniotomy with division of the tentorium, or through a conventional suboccipital craniectomy [11, 12]. While this exposure may be adequate for small tumors, only a combined supra-infratentorial approach offers the wide exposure of the petroclival and bordering areas that is invaluable to deal effectively and safely with the sizeable tumors usually found in this region. In addition to providing wide exposure, a combined supra- and infratentorial approach offers the possibility of attacking the tumors from different angles according to the different stages of the operation. Again, this helps in minimizing the risks to the neurovascular structures. There have been several variations of the combined supra- and infratentorial approach to the petroclival area.

Kempe [6] described an occipital craniotomy combined with a suboccipital craniectomy, opening of the dura above and below the transverse sinus, cutting of the tentorium, and excision of the tumor-alternating a transtentorial removal from above after upward retraction of the occipital lobe with an infratentorial removal from below after medial cerebellar retraction. Malis's [7] version of the combined supra- and infratentorial approach consists of a posterior temporal craniotomy, suboccipital craniectomy, and masteoidectomy. After exposure of the transverse and sigmoid sinus the dura is opened supra- and infratentorially, the transverse sinus is cut distal to the entrance of Labbe's vein and proximal to the sigmoid and superior petrosal sinus. The tentorial margin adherent to the petrous ridge is then transected a few millimeters from the bone to avoid the superior petrosal sinus. The temporal lobe covered by the tentorium is retracted superiorly, while the cerebellum is retracted medially [3, 7]. Al Mefty et al. [1] have recently described a combined supra- and infratentorial petrosal approach to the petroclival area that can be modified into an approach anterior to the sigmoid sinus. Hakuba et al. [4, 5] have described another modification of the combined suprainfratentorial presigmoid approach to the petroclival area that requires a very extensive petrosectomy.

We have recently developed a modification of the combined supra-infratentorial approach which allows for preservation of the transverse sinus while maintaining and even improving the surgical exposure [9]. This approach has rapidly become our approach of choice to the petroclival region because it provides a wide multiangled exposure to the petroclival area while minimizing the amount of temporal lobe, and of cerebellar retraction, preserving at the same time the integrity of the major dural sinuses and the cerebellar parenchyma. The patient lies in the semisitting position with the head carefully flexed and turned 30° toward the side of the lesion. The head is secured by using a three point Mayfield clamp. A curvilinear skin incision starting a few centimeters above and in front of the upper portion of the ear is extended in a linear fashion toward the suboccipital area approximately 1 cm medial to the mastoid process (Fig. 13.1 a). A small temporal craniotomy is performed flush with the base of the middle cranial fossa just anterior to and above the transverse sinus. A suboccipital craniectomy is then executed, exposing the transverse sinus and its junction with the sigmoid sinus. Using a high-speed drill with a carbide bit, an extensive mastoidectomy is carried out with exposure of the full length of the sigmoid sinus as low as the jugular bulb (Fig. 13.1 b).

From now on until the dura is closed the operation is conducted using the operating microscope. The posterior wall of the petrous pyramid is drilled away using a high-speed drill with a diamond bit. The drilling is continued in a lateromedial direction up to the porus acusticus and as far as possible in a posteroanterior direction without entering the bony labyrinth or the fallopian canal. The dura is then incised in an L-shaped fashion with the short limb lying supratentorially just above and lateral to the transverse sinus and the long branch being infratentorially anterior to the sigmoid sinus and extending inferiorly to the jugular bulb (Fig. 13.1 b). The lateral cerebellomedullary cisters is opened, and cerebrospinal fluid is withdrawn to provide extra space. Should the cistern be occluded by tumor, one may tap the occipital horn, open the cisterna magna, or rapidly debulk the tumor. After coagulation of the superior petrosal sinus the tentorial margin adherent to it is transected anteriorly toward the petrous apex. The tentorium is also transected in a lateromedial direction, fashioning a triangularly shaped tentorial flap with its curved base medially toward the incisura and its apex laterally toward the petrous ridge. The occipitotemporal lobe covered by the tentorium is then retracted superiorly while the sigmoid sinus, the cerebellum, and the lateral part of the transverse sinus are retracted medially (Fig. 13.1 c). Great care is necessary not to put tension on Labbe's vein while retracting the occipitotemporal lobe.

Once the meningioma is exposed, it is removed, alternating intratumoral decompression using the ultrasonic aspirator and/or bipolar coagulation and microscissors, with dissection of the tumor from the surrounding structures. To minimize the risk to the neurovascular structures it is imperative to maintain the dissection outside of the arachnoid. While in small petroclival meningiomas the VII-VIII nerve complex is usually easily identifiable on the posterior aspect of the tumor, in large tumors this complex and the lower cranial nerves are engulfed by the tumor, and meticulous microsurgical dissection is necessary to preserve function. We have noted that occasionally these tumors are firmly adherent to the pia at the level of the brainstem, and if an attempt is made to remove this part of the tumor, the pia glia is literaly peeled off from the brainstem, with associated neural injury. In these cases we prefer to be content with a subtotal tumor removal. We agree with Yasargil et al. [12] that the basal dura and undersurface of the tentorium may be diffusely infiltrated so that it is difficult to determine exactly the point of dural attachment. In those cases, in which a limited dural invasion was present, the tumor seemed to be coming from the upper clivus or from the medial portion of the posterior pyramid, but a few times it was originating from the tentorium.

At the end of tumor removal hemostasis is carefully secured, the pyramid defect is filled with a free muscle graft and fibrin glue, the mastoid cells are sealed with bone wax, the dura is closed in a watertight fashion with a running suture, and the muscles and skin are closed as usual. A compressive dressing is applied for 7–10 days.

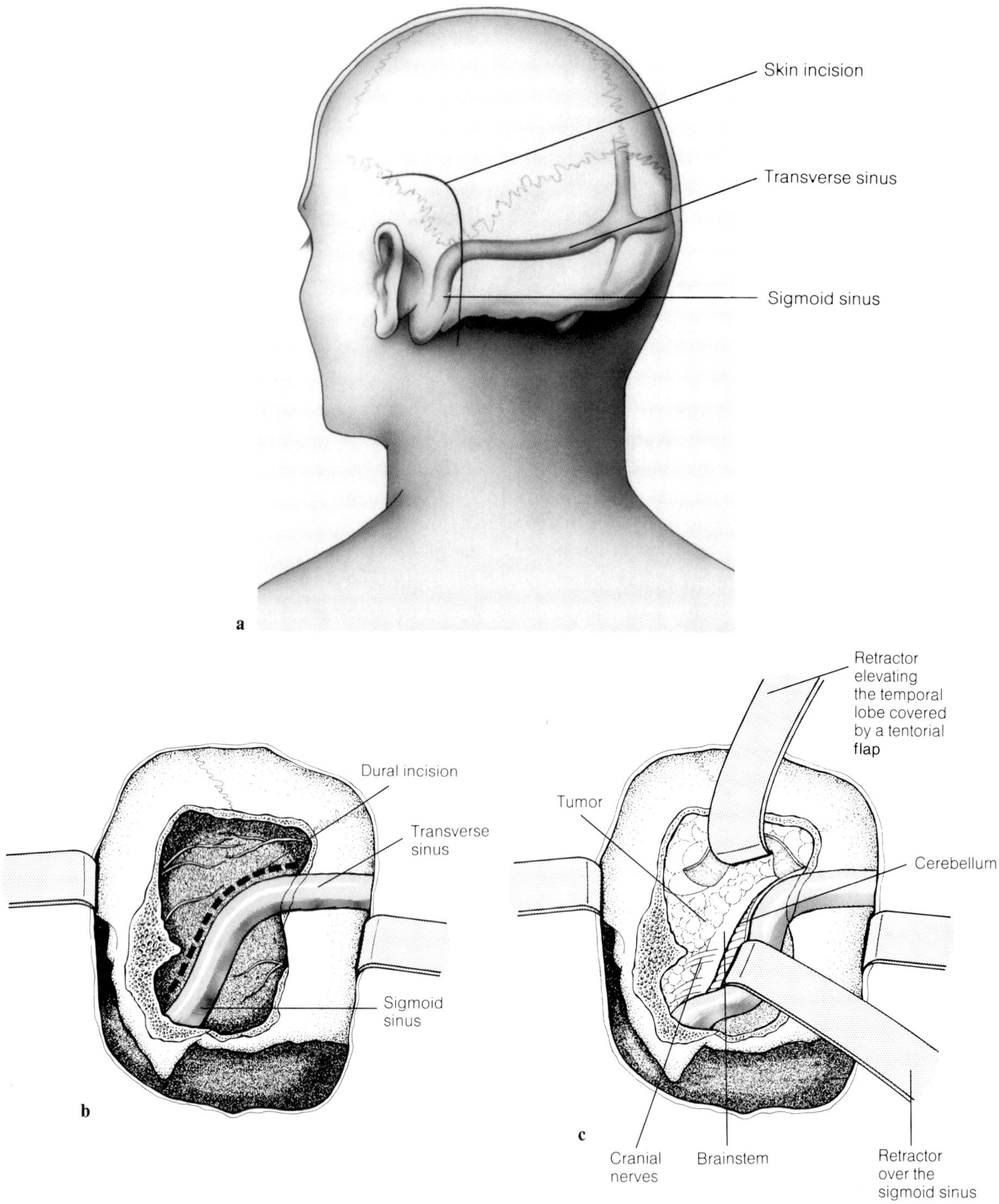

Fig. 13.1 a–c. Diagrammatic representation of the combined supra-infratentorial presigmoid sinus approach to the petroclival region. **a** Skin incision and its relationship to the dural sinuses. **b** Dural incision. **c** Tumor exposure

13.2 a 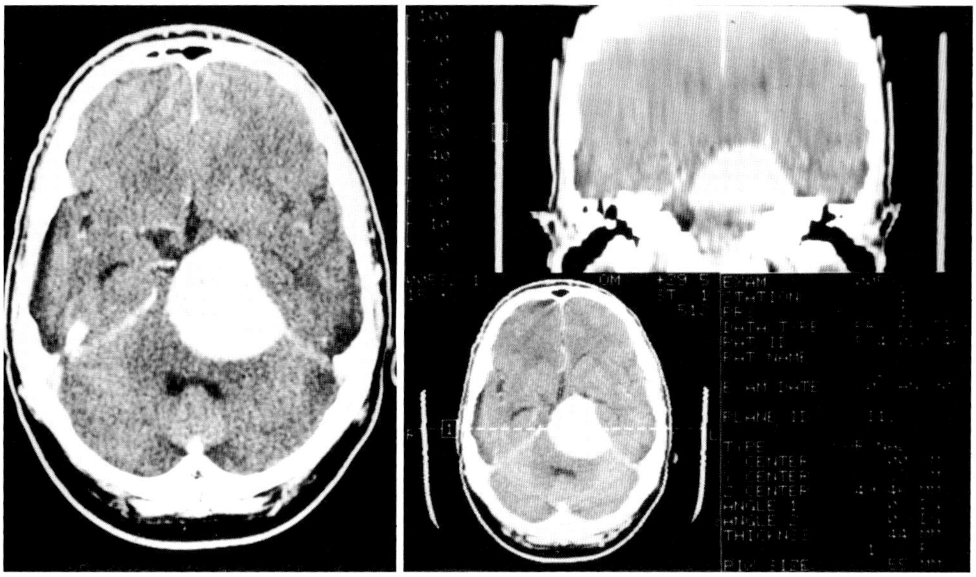 b

13.3 a 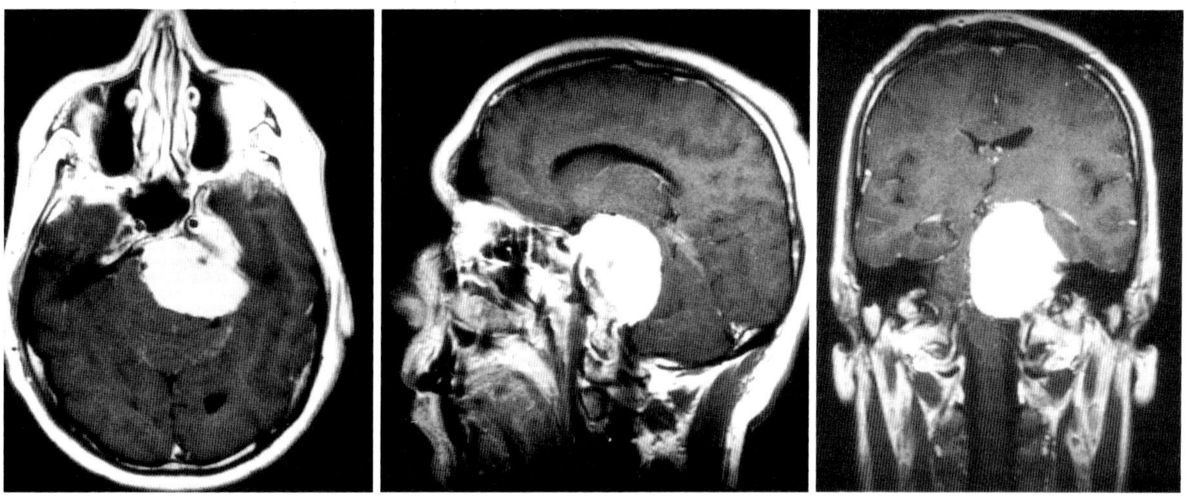 b, c

Illustrative Cases

Case 1. A 44-year-old man presented to us with a 1-year history of decreased hearing on the left and unsteady gait. Neurological examination was positive for a partial facial nerve peripheral paresis on the left, for severely decreased hearing on the left. The gait was unsteady with a broad base, and the cerebellar tests were mildly positive bilaterally. CT and MRI scans showed a large left-sided petroclival tumor extending above the incisura and compressing the brainstem (Figs. 13.2, 13.3). Angiography and xenon CT scans confirmed the tumor hypervascularity (Fig. 13.4). Through a combined supra-

Fig. 13.2 a, b. CT scan of a large petroclival meningioma. **a** Axial enhanced CT scan shows a large tumor in the left petroclival region extending through the incisura to the middle cranial fossa. **b** Axial enhanced CT scan and coronal reconstruction show the large left petroclival tumor and the compressed brainstem

Fig. 13.3 a – c. MRI appearance of petroclival meningioma. **a** Axial gadolinium-enhanced MRI scan shows the tumor engulfment of the left vertebral artery and the relationships between the tumor and the internal carotid artery at the petrous apex. **b** Sagittal gadolinium-enhanced MRI scan demonstrates the caudocranial extent of the tumor and its impingement on the floor of ventricle III. **c** Coronal gadolinium-enhanced MRI scan depicts the tumor deformation of the brainstem and diencephalon

References

1. Al Mefty O, Fox JL, Smith RR (1988) Petrosal approach for petroclival meningiomas. Neurosurgery 22:510–517
2. Castellano F, Ruggiero G (1953) Meningiomas of the posterior fossa. Acta Radiol [Suppl] (Stockh) 104: 1–157
3. Decker RE, Malis LI (1970) Surgical approaches to mid line lesions at the base of the skull: a review. Mt Sinai J Med (NY) 37:84–102
4. Hakuba A, Nishimura S (1981) Total removal of clivus meningiomas and the operative results. Neurol Med Chir 21:59–73
5. Hakuba A, Nishimura S, Jo Jang B (1988) A combined retroauricular and preauricular transpetrosal-transtentorial approach to clivus meningiomas. Surg Neurol 30:108–116
6. Kempe LG (1970) Operative neurosurgery, vol 2. Springer, Berlin Heidelberg New York, pp 45–53
7. Malis LI (1985) Surgical resection of tumours of the skull base. In: Wilkins RH, Rengachary SS (eds) Neurosurgery, vol 1. McGraw-Hill, pp 1011–1021
8. Mayberg MR, Symon LD (1986) Meningiomas of the clivus and apical petrous bone. Report of 35 cases. J Neurosurg 65:160–167
9. Samii M, Ammirati M (1988) The combined supra-infratentorial presigmoid sinus avenue to the petroclival region. Surgical technique and clinical applications. Acta Neurochir (Wien) 95:6–12
10. Samii M, Ammirati M, Mahran A, Bini W, Sephernia A (1989) Surgery of petroclival meningiomas. Report of 24 cases. Neurosurgery 24:12–17
11. Sekhar LN, Samii M (1986) Petroclival and medial tentorial meningiomas. In: Scheunemann H, Schurmann K, Helms J (eds) Tumors of the skull base. Extra- and intracranial surgery of skull base tumours. de Gruyter, Berlin, pp 141–158
12. Yasargil MG, Mortara RW, Curcic M (1980) Meningiomas of basal posterior cranial fossa. In: Krayenbühl H (ed) Advances and technical standards in neurosurgery, vol 7. Springer, Berlin Heidelberg New York, pp 3–115

CHAPTER 14

Incisural Meningiomas

General Considerations

Under the heading of incisural meningiomas we include those tumors presenting in the space between the free edge of the tentorium and the lateral aspect of the cerebral peduncles. This area corresponds to the middle incisura space as described by Ono et al. [4]. Meningiomas of this area may extend anteromedially in the anterior incisura space, anterolaterally in the region of the cavernous sinus and medial middle fossa, laterally over the anterior aspect of the pyramid, inferomedially over the clivus, and inferolaterally in the cerebellopontine angle. These tumors have usually been grouped together with tentorial meningiomas.

Personal Series

Our material is summarized in Table 14.1. One patient was diagnosed because of increased intracranial pressure due to hydrocephalus secondary to aqueductal stenosis resulting from tumor compression; one patient presented with decreased hearing and facial paresis of 1-year duration, one with dizzines and homonymous hemianopia of a few months' duration and, one with a 1-year history of decreased facial sensation, tinnitus, decreased hearing, and unsteady walking. One patient died 1 week postoperatively due to pneumonia without having regained consciousness. Autopsy showed an en plaque meningioma with diffuse infiltration of sphenoid, petrous bone, cavernous sinus, and leptomeninges.

Surgical Considerations

The tumor was approached twice through a frontotemporal and twice through a posterior subtemporal approach. Meningiomas that are mainly located medial to the free edge of the tentorium may be exposed through a frontotemporal transsylvian approach, or through an anterior or posterior subtemporal approach. In the transsylvian approach a curved frontotemporal incision is executed behind the hairline running 1 cm anterior to the tragus (Fig. 14.1). After raising a small frontotemporal

Table 14.1. Incisural meningiomas

Number	4
Age: range/mean/median (years)	46 – 69/54/50.5
Women/men	3/1
Symptom (most common)	Decreased hearing
Sign (most common)	Decreased nerve VII function
Tumor removal	
Total	2
Subtotal	2
Outcome	
Good	2
Fair	1
Poor	0
Deaths	1

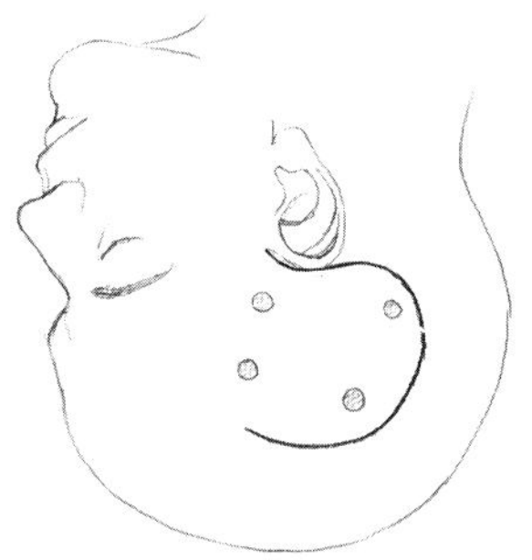

Fig. 14.1. Temporal intradural approach to the middle skull base and tentorial incisura: scalp incision and burrholes

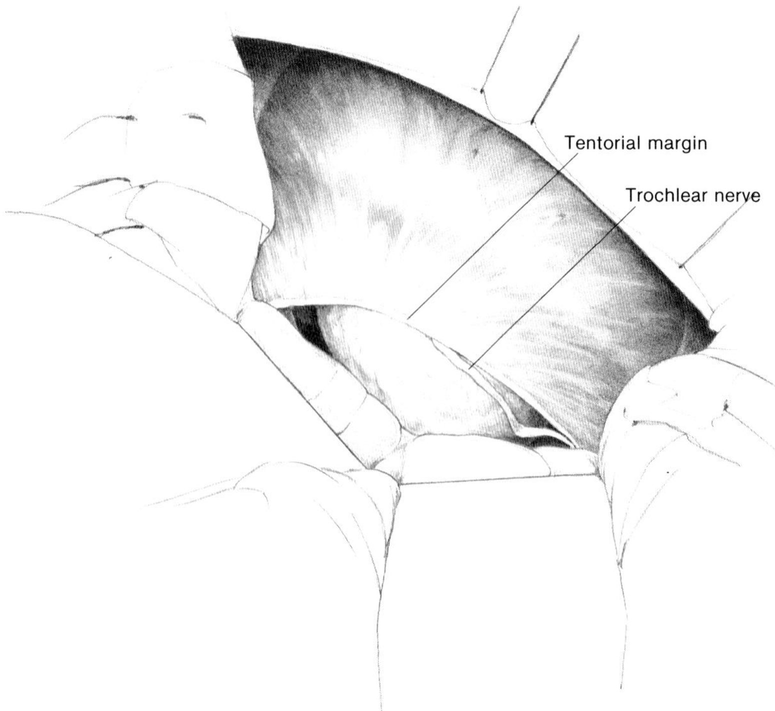

bone flap, removing the lateral part of the lesser sphenoid wing, opening the frontotemporal dura basally, the frontal lobe and the temporal pole are elevated from the anterior and middle fossa using self-retaining retractors. The approach is then continued intradurally along the sphenoid wing in the direction of the anterior clinoid process by gradually opening the cisterns and removing cerebrospinal fluid. This procedure must not be rushed, so that by constant aspiration of cerebrospinal fluid and gentle retraction the frontal and temporal lips of the sylvian fissure can be gradually opened on the frontal lobe side without any undue pressure on the brain.

After exposure of the optic nerve and the further opening of the cisterns along the free tentorial edge, the internal carotid artery, posterior communicating artery, and anterior choroidal artery are exposed in the anterior third of the tentorial notch (Figs. 14.2, 14.3). Nerve III may or may not be evident at this time. The tentorial width is extremely variable [2], and this may influence the surgical strategy. Exposure may be increased by cutting the free edge of the tentorium. This maneuver must be preceded by coagulation of the superior petrosal sinus and identification of the trochlear nerve (Fig. 14.4). Additional exposure may be gained by drilling off the petrous bone between the entrance of the trigeminal nerve into Meckel's cave anteriorly, the anterior wall of the internal auditory canal posteriorly, and the intrapetrous internal carotid artery laterally (Fig. 14.7). The drilling of the petrous apex is a demanding and dangerous surgical task and must always be performed with great caution. The tumor removal is then performed from lateral to medial, toward the brainstem

Fig. 14.2. After incision of the dura, the frontal lobe is retracted anteriorly and the temporal lobe posteromedially to expose the tumor in the tentorial incisura. The trochlear nerve passes over the tumor surface

Fig. 14.3. Further brain retraction uncovers the internal carotid artery and optic nerve anteriorly. The trochlear nerve is very carefully mobilized from the tumor capsule

Fig. 14.4. Further tumor exposure may be gained by cutting across the tentorial margin after bipolar coagulation. Care is taken not to damage the subjacent trochlear nerve

Fig. 14.5. Piecemeal enucleation of the tumor. The oculomotor nerve is visible deep in the field

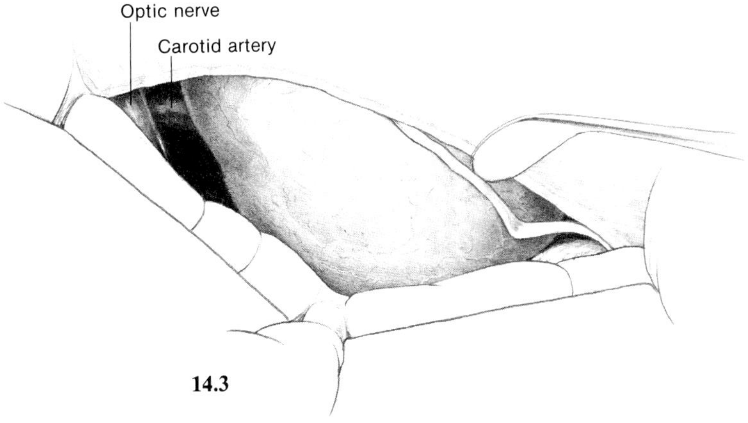
Optic nerve
Carotid artery

14.3

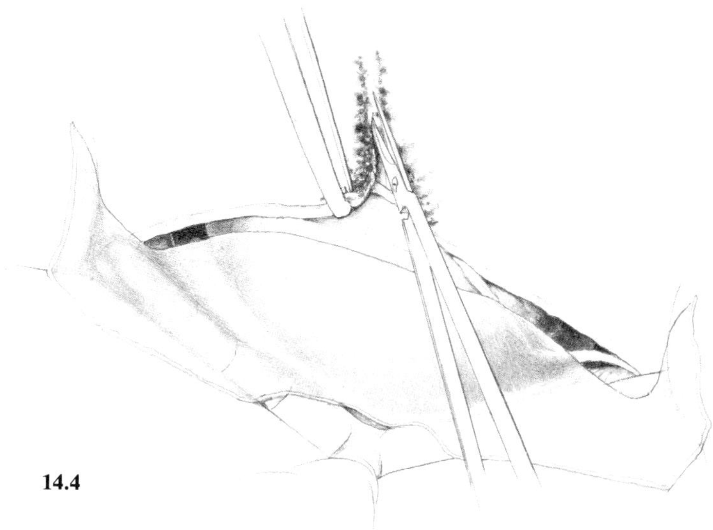

14.4

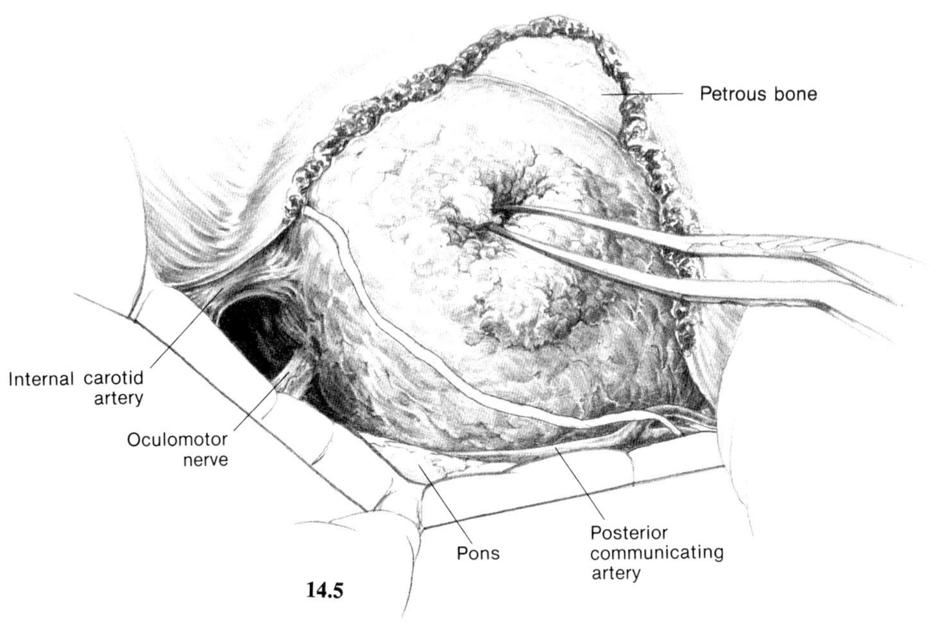
Petrous bone
Internal carotid artery
Oculomotor nerve
Pons
Posterior communicating artery

14.5

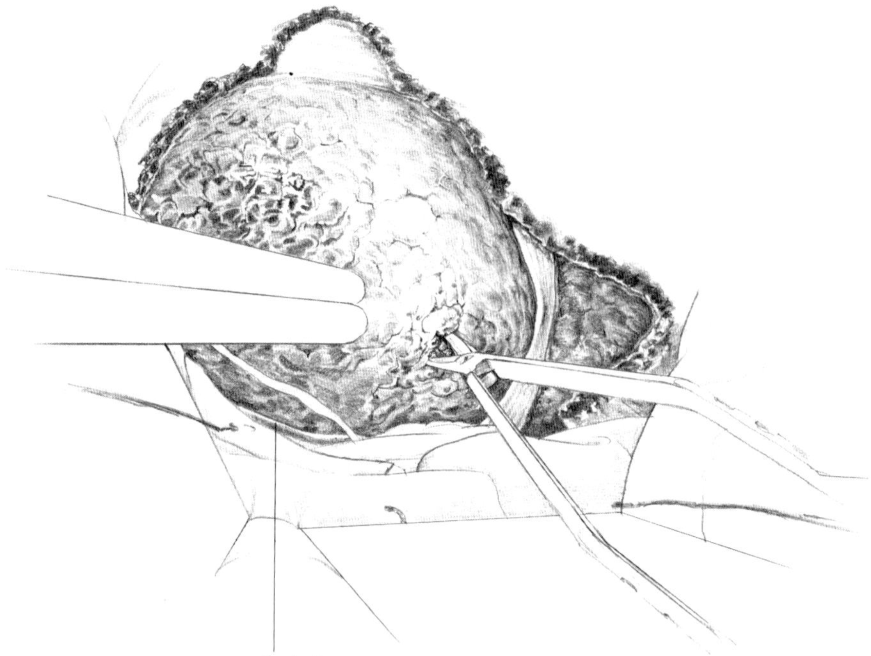

14.6

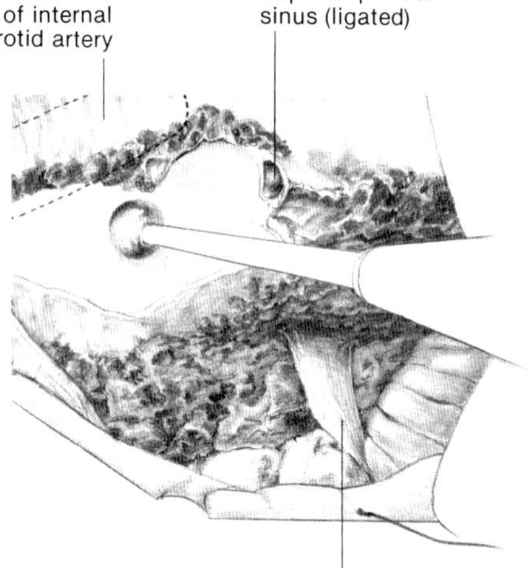

14.7

Fig. 14.6. As tumor removal is carried further posteriorly, the trigeminal nerve comes into view

Fig. 14.7. The view into the cerebellopontine angle is facilitated by drilling away the medial part of the petrous apex. This is done after coagulation and division of the superior petrosal sinus and resection of the dura covering the pyramidal surface

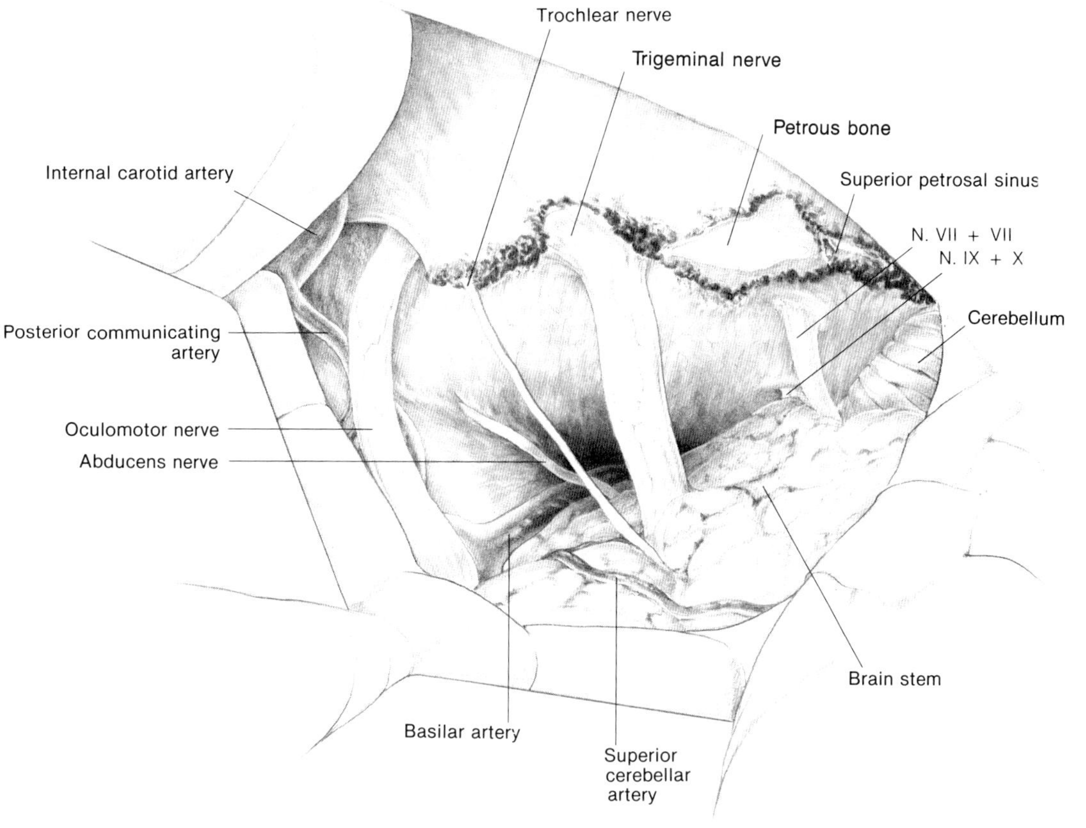

Fig. 14.8. Appearance of the surgical cavity at the end of the procedure. Brain and neurovascular structures have been preserved

(Figs. 14.5 – 14.8). This part of the procedure is complicated by the intimate relationships between the tumor and perforating vessels to the brainstem. We believe that those vessels supplying the tumor and the brainstem may be transected if they need to be; it seems more dangerous to apply traction to brainstem vessels by pulling on the tumor. However, transection of these vessels should not be done lightly because it is not possible to predict the exact effect of any individual vessel transection [3]. Using this exposure, the middle incisural space is approached along an anteroposterior plane lateral to the supraclinoid internal carotid artery.

The anterior subtemporal approach differs from the transsylvian because the sylvian fissure is not opened. The skin incision is placed slightly more posteriorly than the one previously described. The middle incisural space is always approached along an anteroposterior plane but more laterally coming from underneath the temporal lobe. At times the temporal pole is already partially elevated from the middle fossa floor by the tumor [5].

The skin incision used for the posterior subtemporal approach resembles a reverse question mark starting in front of the tragus. A posterior temporal craniotomy combined with a low basal temporal craniectomy is then executed and the basal temporal dura opened. The temporal lobe is then retracted superiorly and the middle incisural space reached; the tentorium needs to be incised, always posterior to nerve IV, and great care must be used not to injure this nerve. The posterior subtemporal avenue is the most direct approach to the middle incisural space, which is reached in a straight lateral direction. Its main drawbacks is the temporal lobe retraction with its associated sequelae. The amount of temporal lobe retraction may be somewhat reduced by early and wide opening of the cisterns, if not occupied by the tumor. A lumbar subarachnoid catheter may also be used to this effect.

a b c d
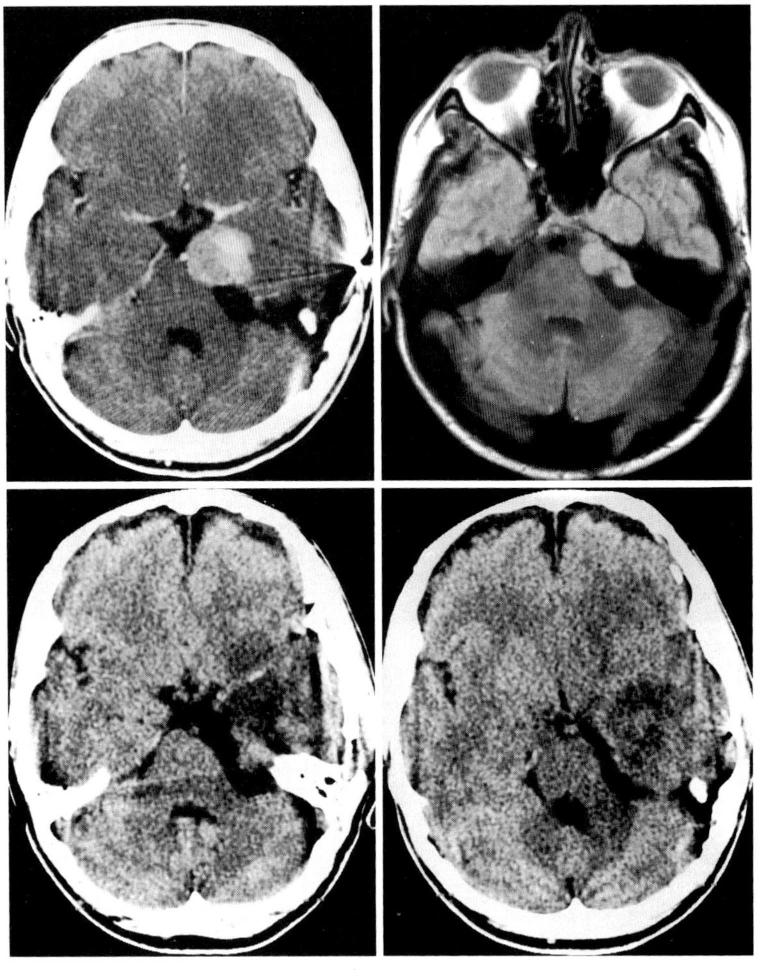

Fig. 14.9 a–d. A 52-year-old woman with left incisural meningioma. **a, b** Preoperative CT and MRI scans show the left incisural meningioma. **c, d** Postoperative CT scans show total tumor removal

The choice among these approaches depends on the direction of growth of the tumor. For a tumor limited to the middle incisural space a posterior subtemporal approach is probably adequate, while for a tumor extending anteriorly from this space to involve the cavernous sinus and the medial middle fossa, a frontotemporal transsylvian or anterior subtemporal approach or a combination of the two would be preferable.

Illustrative Case

A 52-year-old woman had been complaining for the past few years of generalized headache. An incisural meningioma was eventually diagnosed, and she was operated on elsewhere through a temporo-occipital approach that failed to remove the whole tumor. At the time of her presentation to us she showed negative neurological examination results, and a left incisural meningioma was demonstrated by CT and MRI scans (Fig. 14.9a, b). Through a frontotemporal craniotomy with wide opening of the sylvian fissure an incisural supra-infratentorial meningioma extending into the posterior portion of the cavernous sinus and around the basilar artery was completely removed with preservation of all cranial nerves. The postoperative course was uneventful, and she was discharged with no neurological deficit. Postoperative CT scan confirmed total tumor removal (Fig. 14.2c, d).

References

1. Guidetti B, Ciappetta P, Domenicucci M (1988) Tentorial meningiomas: surgical experience with 61 cases and long term results. J Neurosurg 69:183–187
2. Lang J (1985) Anatomy of the tentorial margin. Adv Neurosurg 13:173–182
3. Mitterwallner FV (1955) Variationsstatistische Untersuchungen an den basalen Hintergefäßen. Acta Anat (Basel) 24:51–70
4. Ono M, Ono M, Rhoton AL, Barry M (1984) Microsurgical anatomy of the region of the tentorial incisura. J Neurosurg 60:365–399
5. Sekhar LN, Jannetta PJ (1987) Petroclival and medial tentorial meningiomas. In: Sekhar LN, Schramm VL Jr (eds) Tumors of the cranial base: diagnosis and treatment. Futura, Mount Kisko, pp 623–640
6. Sekhar LN, Jannetta PJ, Maroon JC (1984) Tentorial meningiomas. Surgical management and results. Neurosurgery 14:268–275

CHAPTER 15

Trigeminal Meningiomas

General Considerations

Meningiomas originating in Meckel's cave represent, together with neurinomas, the most common lesion found in this area. According to Butti et al. neurinomas of Meckel's cave outnumber meningiomas almost 3 to 1 [2]. Clinically these tumors present with typical or atypical trigeminal neuralgia. The location of trigeminal meningiomas with respect to the ganglion or roots does not help to shed light on the mechanisms of trigeminal neuralgia. In a recent report two out of four patients with trigeminal meningiomas had trigeminal neuralgia, and both of them had tumors compressing the trigeminal roots in the upper cerebellopontine angle [1]; however, there are many other reports of typical or atypical trigeminal neuralgia associated with tumors confined to Meckel's cave [3, 4]. Before the advent of CT many of these meningiomas were discovered incidentally during surgery for retrogasserian rhizothomy.

Personal Series

Table 15.1 shows our material. Of our four patients, two presented with typical trigeminal neuralgia of 1- and 4-years' duration, respectively, and negative results on neurological examination; one with a 1-year history of exophthalmos and double vision and with a partial nerve III paresis; and the last one presented with a 3-year history of decreased hearing and a 2-month history of cerebellar symptoms with decreased facial sensation, decreased hearing, decreased lower cranial nerve (IX-XI) function, and positive cerebellar tests. In the two patients with trigeminal neuralgia the tumor was in the cave in one and in the upper cerebellopontine angle in the other; in the patient with exophthalmos it extended into the cavernous sinus, and in the one with an acoustic-like history the tumor was extending into the cerebellopontine angle.

Surgical Considerations

The tumor was approached through a lateral suboccipital craniectomy in the two cases in which it presented mainly in the cerebellopontine angle and through a frontotemporal transsylvian route when it was located mainly in the middle fossa. Two of the four tumors extended en plaque from the cave and were subtotally removed, while two with a globular type of growth were totally removed.

Illustrative Cases

Case 1. A 56-year-old woman presented with a 3-year history of decreased hearing and a 2-month history of unsteady gait and trouble in swallowing. Neurological examination was positive for mildly

Table 15.1. Trigeminal meningiomas

Number	4
Age: range/mean/median (years)	46 – 71/57/55
Women/men	4/0
Symptom (most common)	Facial pain
Sign (most common)	Decreased nerve V function
Tumor removal	
Total	2
Subtotal	2
Outcome	
Good	3
Fair	0
Poor	1
Deaths	0

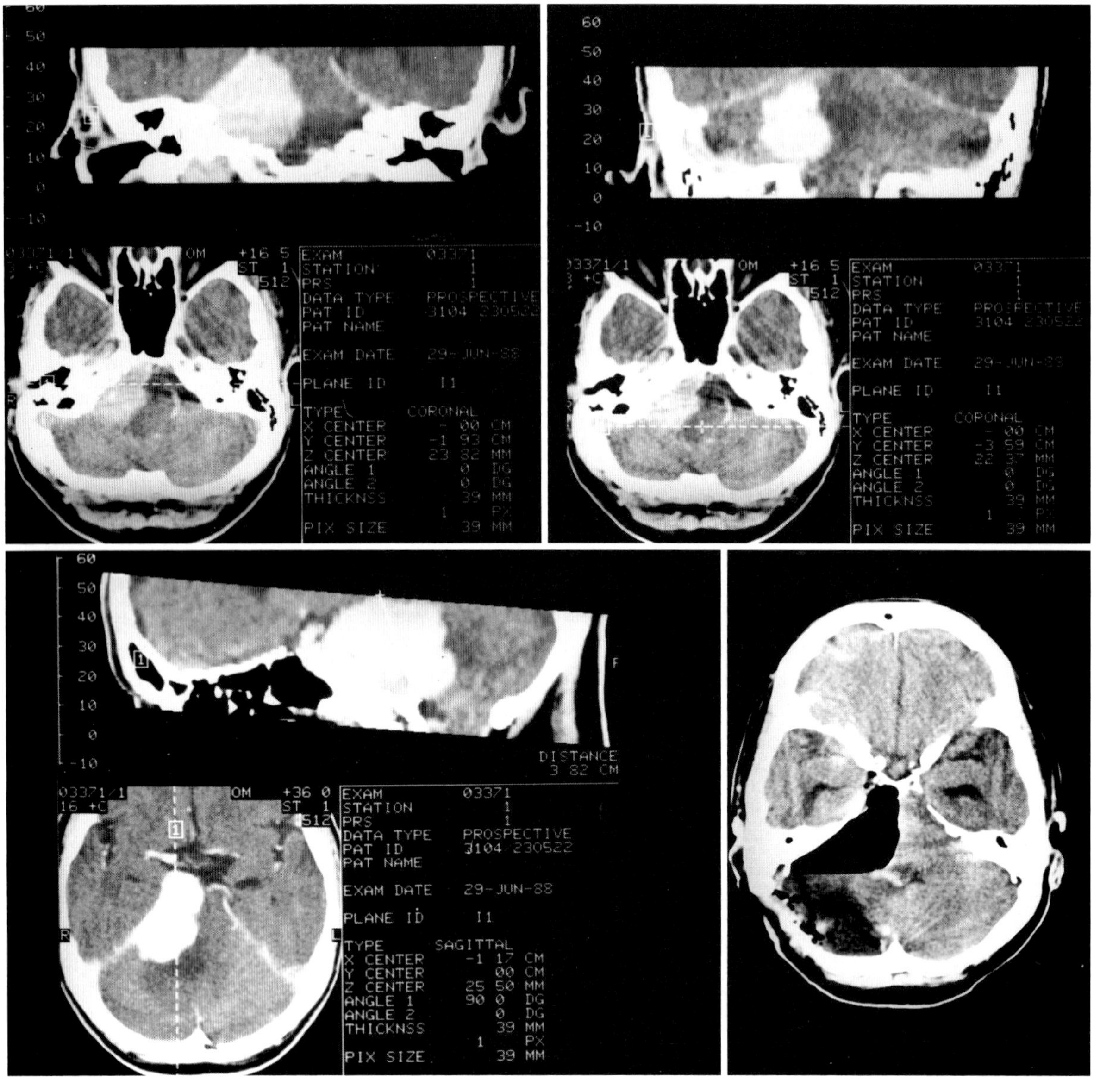

a b c d

Fig. 15.1 a–d. A 56-year-old woman with cerebellar findings and large right trigeminal meningioma. CT scans show a large meningioma. The relationship of the tumor to the tentorium and to the skull base are well depicted in the coronal (**a, b**) and sagittal (**c**) reconstructions. **d** Postoperative CT scan shows total tumor removal

decreased sensation over the left face, decreased hearing, decreased IX-XI nerve function, and positive cerebellar tests were. CT scans showed a 5-cm tumor in the cerebellopontine angle with severe degree of cerebellar-brainstem edema (Fig. 15.1 a–c). At surgery, by suboccipital craniectomy, a tumor originating from the posterior fossa opening of Meckel's cave, displacing the nerve VII-VIII complex dorsally and the cranial nerves IX-XI caudally was completely removed. Nerve V was invaded by tumor and had to be sacrificed. Due to difficulties in waking up from the anesthesia a CT scan was obtained, which showed a cerebellar blood clot in the area of preoperative swelling, compressing the IV ventricle with hydrocephalus. The hematoma was removed, and the patient was discharged 3 months after the operation, awake, following commands, with a left hemiparesis. Postoperative CT scan showed total tumor removal (Fig. 15.1 d). We have also seen this intracerebellar intra brainstem bleeding a few other times in the area of the preoperative swelling after the removal of large cerebellopontine angle tumors. We think this may represent a relatively sudden perfusion of areas that were chronically underperfused for a long time and whose blood flow control mechanism are probably dysregulated. A long period (1 week to 10 days) of antiedema treatment and/or a planned two-stage surgical procedure could reduce the occurrence of this complication.

Case 2. A 54-year-old woman came to us for microvascular decompression due to a 4-year history of trigeminal neuralgia resistant to medical treatment and to thermocoagulation, which had been tried twice before. Neurological examination was negative. CT scans showed a cerebellopontine angle tumor. By a lateral suboccipital craniectomy a tumor coming from Meckel's cave and pushing nerve V and the nerve VII-VIII complex caudally was completely removed. The postoperative course was uncomplicated, and the patient was sent home on no medication and was pain-free.

References

1. Beck DW, Menezes AH (1987) Lesions in Meckel's cave: variable presentation and pathology. J Neurosurg 67:684–689
2. Butti G, Gaetani P, Giordana MT, Paoletti P (1983) Meningiomas of Meckel's cave. Surg Neurol 20:305–309
3. Nager GT (1984) Neurinomas of the trigeminal nerve. Am J Otolaryngol 5:301–333
4. Nijensahn DE, Araujo JC, MacCarty CS (1975) Meningiomas of Meckel's cave. J Neurosurg 43:197–202

CHAPTER 16

Meningiomas Involving the Cavernous Sinus

General and Surgical Considerations

Surgery of the cavernous sinus has received great impetus in the past few years [3, 9], and its indications are still being defined [9]. Dolenc et al. [3] have reported 63 patients who underwent neoplastic intracavernous surgery, 40 of whom for meningiomas, with an overall mortality rate of 6%, permanent cranial nerve (II-VI) morbidity of 22%, and a total tumor removal of 71% and 73% of the patients returning to their premorbid activity. Sekhar et al. [9] were able totally to remove 13 of 17 (76%) intracavernous meningiomas, and in 42 patients undergoing intracavernous operations for neoplasms there was no mortality; extraocular muscle function was worse in 12%, better in 42%, and unchanged in 69%, and most of the patients had a good performance score postoperatively. Kawase et al. [5] reported on total removal of 5/7 intracavernous meningiomas, with two patients experiencing permanent cranial nerve worsening. The majority of meningiomas reported by Dolenc et al. [3], Sekhar et al. [9] and Kawase et al. [5] were invading the cavernous sinus from surrounding areas. Lesoin et al. [7], reporting on 16 patients with purely intracavernous meningiomas stated that total removal of intracavernous meningiomas is not possible without permanently jeopardizing cranial nerve function. It is evident that removal of intracavernous meningiomas is more dangerous than removal of intracavernous neurinomas or chondromas [7, 9].

The cavernous sinus may be invaded by middle fossa meningiomas, such as sphenoid wing meningiomas, by incisural or trigeminal meningiomas, and by clival, petroclival, or posterior pyramid meningiomas [3, 5]. While we have been very aggressive in removing intracavernous extensions coming from a globular type of tumor when it was evident that removal of this part of the tumor would have resulted in a surgical cure, we have not been equally aggressive in entering the cavernous sinus when it was invaded by an en plaque type of tumor, such as some medial sphenoid wing meningiomas and some medial incisural meningiomas. In these instances invasion of the cavernous sinus is only part of a generalized type of tumor growth that usually diffusely involves the medial cranial base and may even involve, through the neurovascular foramina, the extradural space at the level of the inferior skull base. We believe that these type of tumors are not surgically curable; removing the intracavernous portion of the tumor increases morbidity and still does not cure the patient; furthermore removal of the intracavernous internal carotid artery and bypass between the intrapetrous and the supraclinoidal internal carotid artery is rarely if ever indicated. Radiation therapy has been shown to be effective in the treatment of meningiomas and is therefore a reasonable option in such cases [1, 2, 8]. However, considering that the biological behavior of an individual meningioma is not known, and that radiation therapy has its own risks, we have generally followed up these patients with regularly spaced CT or MRI scans and have recommended radiation therapy when there was neuroradiological or clinical evidence of tumor progression. If the tumor progresses despite radiation therapy, a salvage type of surgical procedure may be considered, and the morbidity that may be associated with it is better understood by the patient and by the surgeon who knows that nothing else could have been done.

In cases of involvement of the cavernous sinus by a globular, not en plaque, type of tumor we have been led into the cavernous sinus by the tumor. Using careful microsurgical technique, it is usually possible to remove the tumor without injuring the intracavernous carotid artery or cranial nerves.

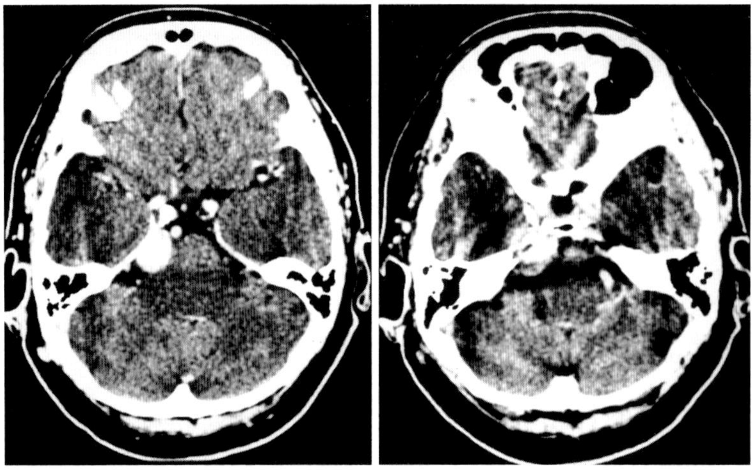

16.1a b

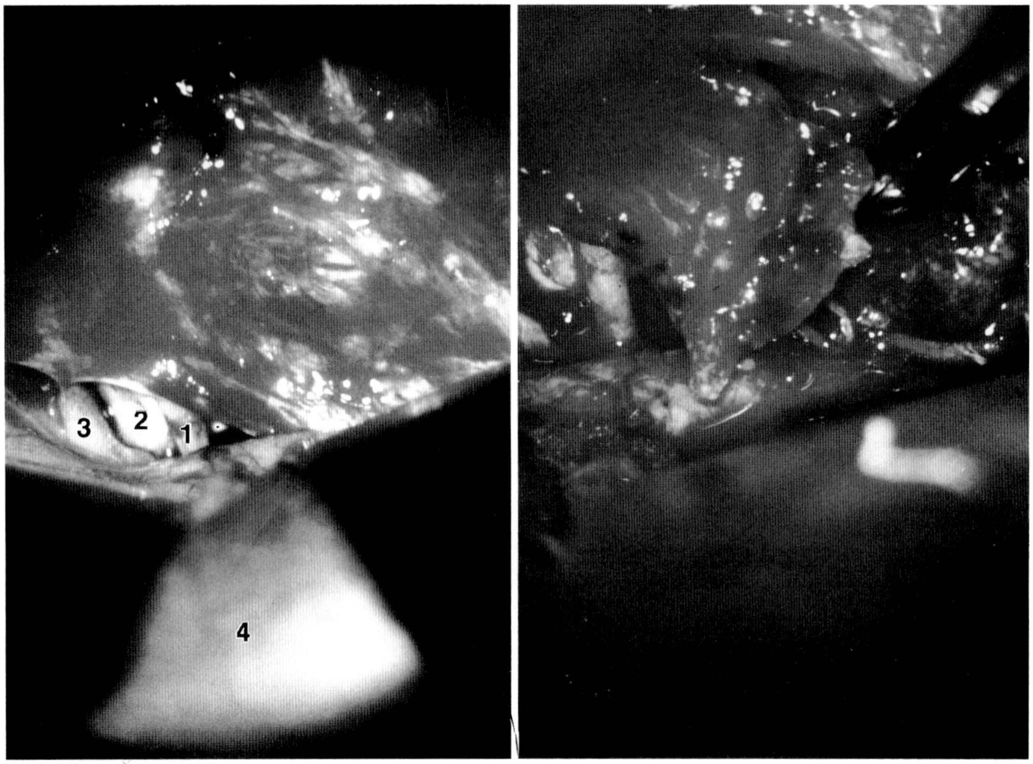

16.2a b

Brisk venous bleeding confirms that the tumor has been removed. This bleeding may be relatively easily controlled by packing the sinus with Gelfoam, Surgicel, or muscle and eventually suturing the dura over the defect. If the dura has been widely excised, a piece of muscle or lyodura held in place with fibrin glue may be used. Such cases have been encountered not infrequently in posterior pyramid, petroclival, and incisural meningiomas and have not been counted here among cavernous sinus me-

Fig. 16.1a, b. Incisural meningioma extending into the cavernous sinus, approached through a frontotemporal transsylvian route. Preoperative axial CT scans show the incisural meningioma invading the cavernous sinus

Fig. 16.2a. Superolateral view of posterior cavernous sinus bulging with tumor. *1*, Oculomotor nerve; *2*, posterior clinoid process; *3*, internal carotid artery; *4*, retractor on temporal lobe. **b** The cavernous sinus has been opened posterior to the nerve IV entrance, and tumor is being removed from inside the cavernous sinus

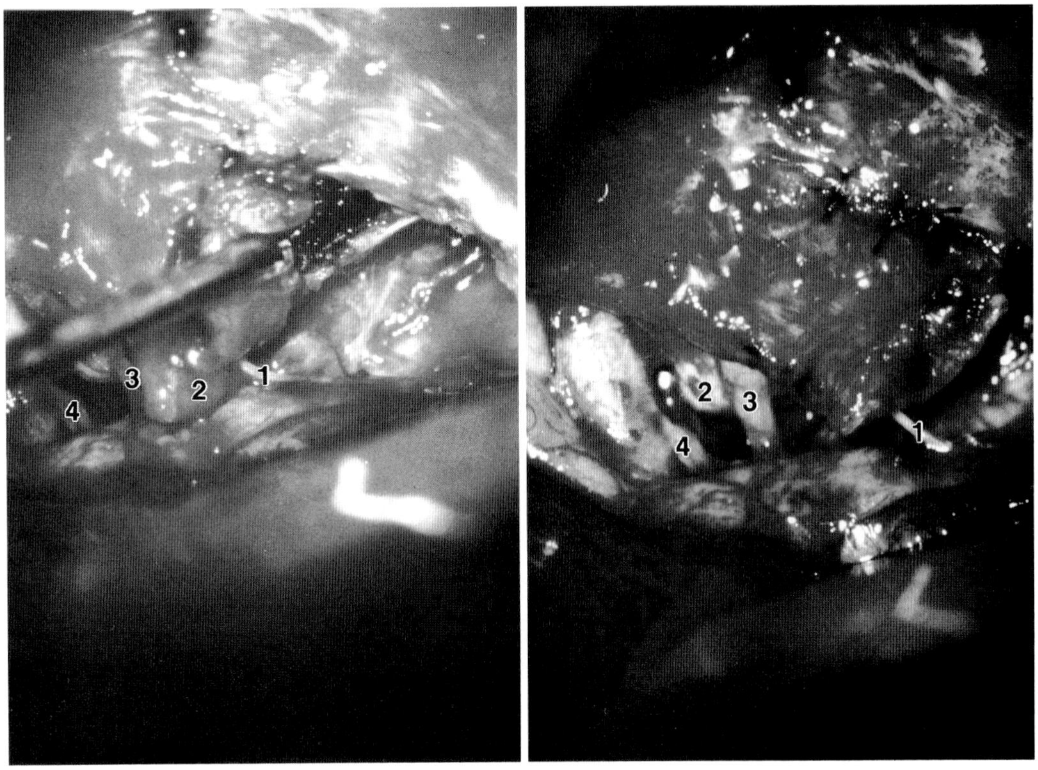

16.3 a b

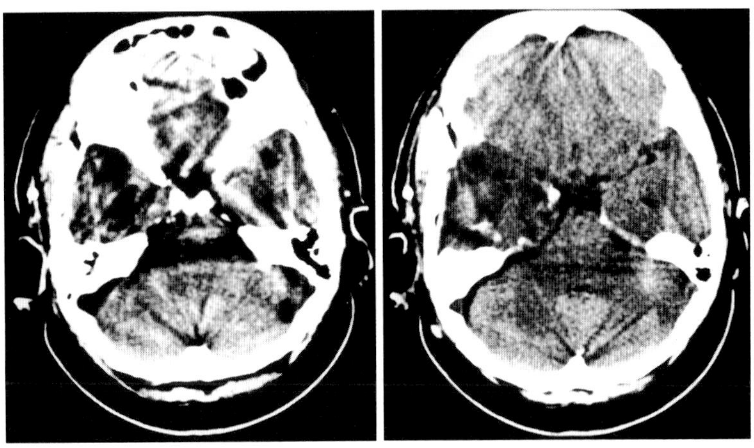

16.4 a b

Fig. 16.3. **a** After tumor removal, Surgicel is being packed inside the cavernous sinus. **b** The cavernous sinus has been packed with Surgicel and the dura over it has been sutured. The oculomotor and trochlear nerves have been preserved. *1*, Trochlear nerve; *2*, posterior clinoid process; *3*, oculomotor nerve; *4*, posterior communicating artery

Fig. 16.4 a, b. Postoperative axial CT scans show total tumor removal

ningiomas because the cavernous sinus was secondarily involved by the tumor. One such a case, that of an incisural meningioma extending into the cavernous sinus is presented in Figs. 16.1 – 16.4.

Meningiomas arising primarily in the cavernous sinus and diagnosed very early, when their intracavernous origin may be easily determined, are very rare. In these instances the possibility of a surgical cure might exist, although meningiomas originating in or invading the cavernous sinus may invade

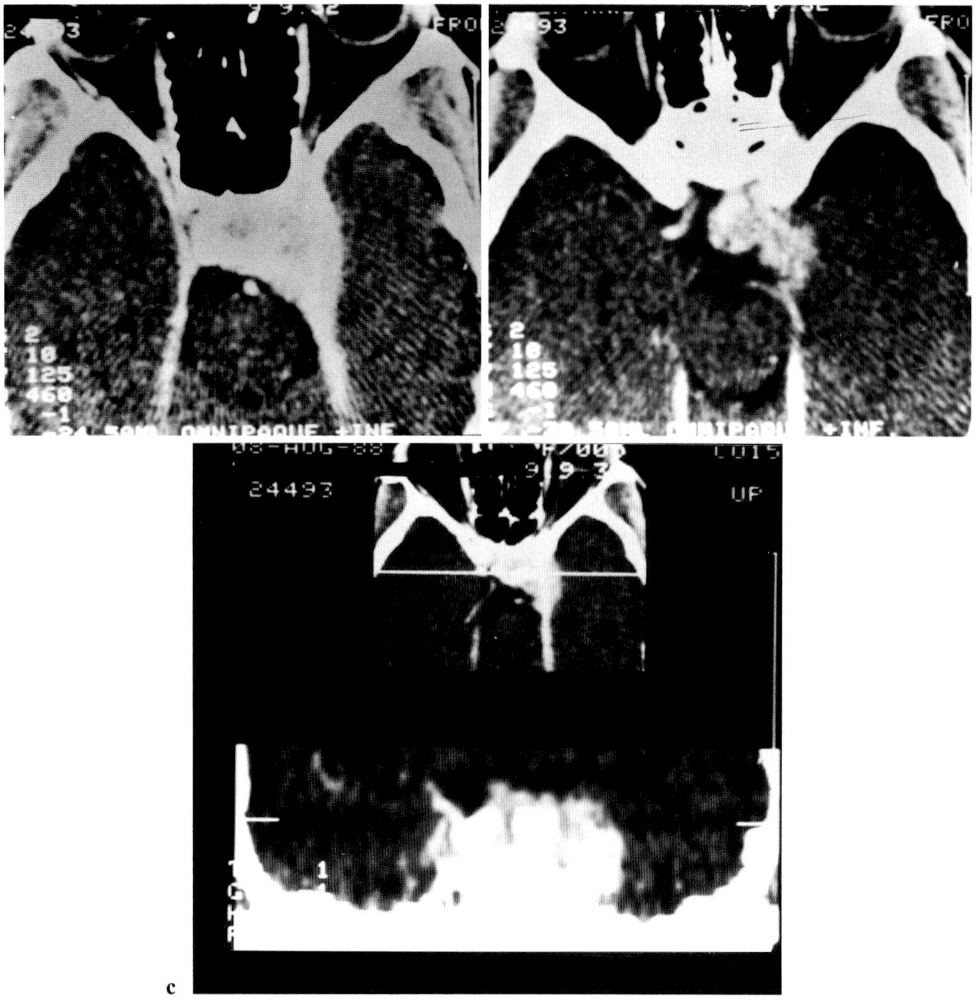

Fig. 16.5 a – c. A 50-year-old woman with intracavernous tumor, probably a meningioma, whose cranial nerve deficits resolved upon discontinuation of estroprogestin medications. Surgery was not performed. **a, b** Axial CT scans show the enhancing intracavernous lesion invading the upper clivus and the petrous apex. **c** Coronal CT reconstruction suggests spread to the contralateral cavernous sinus

Table 16.1. Cavernous sinus meningiomas

Number	1
Age (years)	49
Women/men	0/1
Symptom (most common)	Seizures (see text)
Sign (most common)	None
Tumor removal	
Total	1
Subtotal	0
Outcome	
Good	1
Fair	0
Poor	0
Deaths	0

the contralateral cavernous sinus through the connective tissue strands connecting the two cavernous sinuses [6]. This small group of patients should be given the option of an operation in the understanding that the natural history of meningiomas in this location is unknown. We examined a 50-year-old postmenopausal woman who had been complaining of headache and nerve III and VI paresis. Her CT scans showed a small left-sided intracavernous tumor, probably a meningioma, already spreading to the upper clivus, the petrous apex, and possibly the contralateral cavernous sinus (Fig. 16.5); her symptoms disappeared upon withholding her estroprogestin preparations. Among our 261 skull base meningiomas a meningioma originating and confined to the cavernous sinus was seen only once.

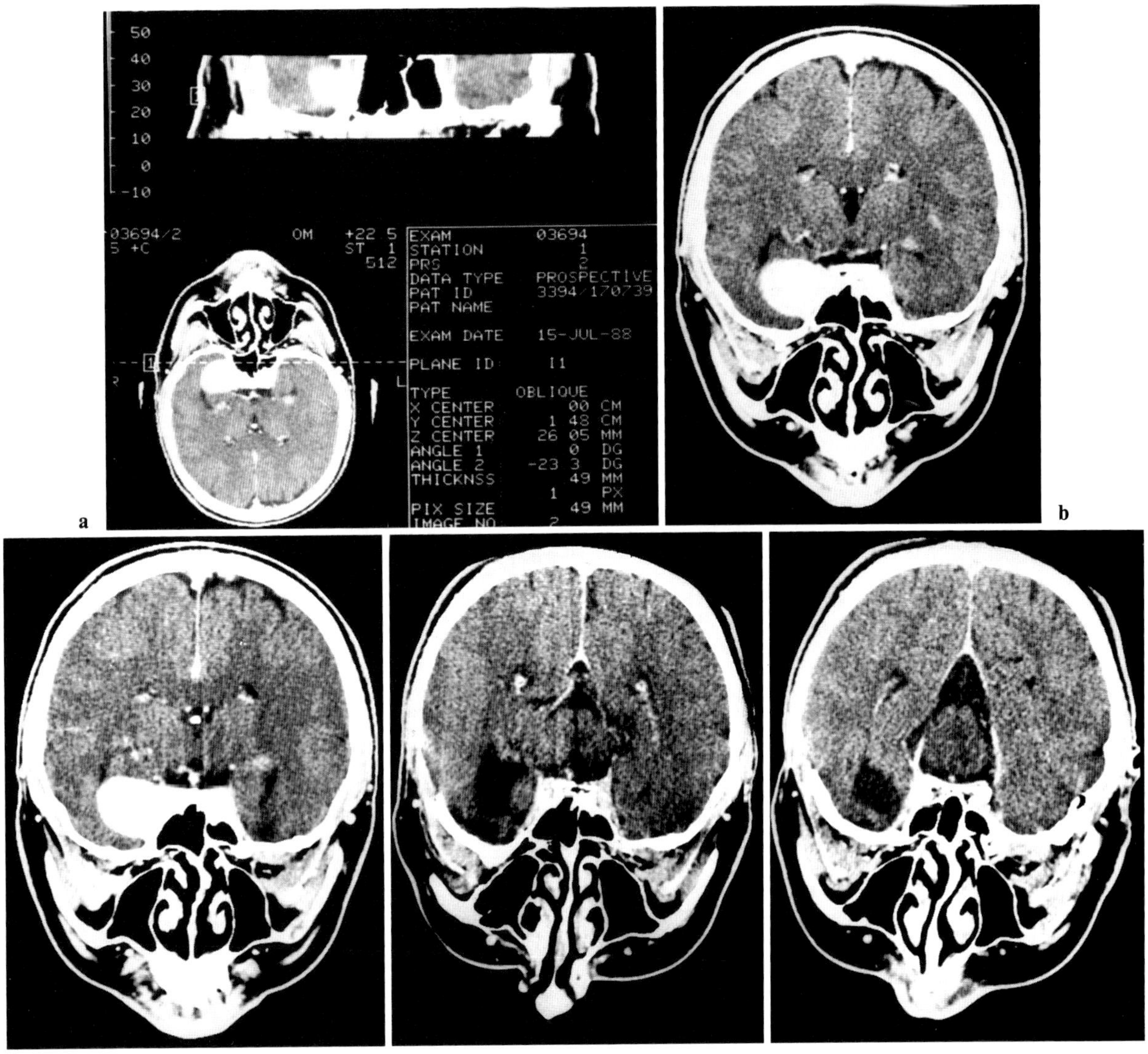

a b c, d e

Fig. 16.6 a–e. A 49-year-old man with temporal lobe seizures and pure intracavernous meningioma. Axial (**a**) and coronal (**b, c**) CT scans show this rare globular type of meningioma exclusively confined to the cavernous sinus. **d, e** Postoperative enhanced coronal CT scans show total tumor removal

This case is described in detail below (see "Illustrative Case"). It is also presented in Table 16.1.

A variety of surgical approaches tailored to the cavernous sinus have been described in the past few years [4, 9]; in our series the surgical approach to tumors invading the cavernous sinus was dictated by the location of the main tumor bulk while the tumor confined to the cavernous sinus was approached through a frontotemporal transsylvian route.

Illustrative Case

A 49-year-old man came to our attention with a diagnosis of cavernous sinus tumor. The tumor had been discovered during work-up of temporal lobe epilepsy. He had a negative neurological examination. He was offered the option of surgery, and by a frontotemporal transsylvian craniotomy the cavernous sinus was exposed, seen to be bulging, opened superior to V1 and intracavernous tumor totally removed. Postoperatively the patient had a transient nerve III and VI paresis. Pre- and postoperative CT scans are shown in Fig. 16.6.

References

1. Barbaro NM, Gutin PH, Wilson CB, Sheline GE, Boldrey EB, Wara WM (1987) Radiation therapy in the treatment of partially resected meningiomas. Neurosurgery 20:525–528
2. Carella RJ, Ransohoff J, Newall J (1982) Role of radiation therapy in the management of meningiomas. Neurosurgery 10:332–339
3. Dolenc VV, Kregar T, Ferluga M, Fettich M, Morina A (1987) Treatment of tumors invading the cavernous sinus. In: Dolenc VV (ed) The cavernous sinus. A multidisciplinary approach to tumorous and vascular lesions. Springer, Berlin Heidelberg New York, pp 377–391
4. Inoue T, Rhoton AL, Theele D, Barry ME (1990) Surgical approaches to the cavernous sinus: a microsurgical study. Neurosurgery 26:903–932
5. Kawase T, Toya S, Shiobara R, Kimura C, Nakajima H (1987) Skull base approaches for meningiomas invading the cavernous sinus. In: Dolenc VV (ed) The cavernous sinus. A multidisciplinary approach to tumorous and vascular lesions. Springer, Berlin Heidelberg New York, pp 346–354
6. Krivosic I, Jomin M, Christiaens JC, Lesoin F, Combelles G, Pruvoj P, Reyford M, Dupont A (1987) Pathological aspects in a series of 53 cavernous sinus tumors. In: Dolenc VV (ed) The cavernous sinus. A multidisciplinary approach to tumorous and vascular lesions. Springer, Berlin Heidelberg New York, pp 392–396
7. Lesoin F, Pellerin P, Autricque A, Clarisse J, Jomin M (1987) The direct microsurgical approach to intracavernous tumors. In: Dolenc VV (ed) The cavernous sinus. A multidisciplinary approach to tumorous and vascular lesions. Springer, Berlin Heidelberg New York, pp 323–331
8. Petty AM, Kun LE, Meyer GA (1985) Radiation therapy for incompletely resected meningiomas. J Neurosurg 62:502–507
9. Sekhar LN, Sen CN, Jho HD, Janecka IP (1989) Surgical treatment of intracavernous neoplasms: a four year experience. Neurosurgery 24:18–30

CHAPTER 17

Meningiomas in Miscellaneous Locations

Personal Series

We have had nine patients with tumors in miscellaneous locations: two coming from the lateral floor of the middle fossa; one in the temporal squama, middle and inner ear extending en plaque intradurally; one in the anteromedial frontal basis going into the sphenoid and frontal sinus; one in the petrous pyramid and cerebellopontine angle; one in ventricle IV and cerebellopontine angle; one en plaque in the anterior, middle, and posterior fossa; one involving the anterior and middle skull base bilaterally and the posterior fossa on one side; and one in the petrous pyramid, temporo-occipital bone, and cerebellopontine angle. The last of these is described in detail below ("Illustrative Case"). Table 17.1 details our material.

Table 17.1. Meningiomas in miscellaneous locations

Number	9
Age: range/mean/median (years)	19–66/42/49
Women/men	3/6
Symptom (most common)	See text
Sign (most common)	See text
Tumor removal	
Total	6
Subtotal	3
Outcome	
Good	7
Fair	1
Poor	1
Deaths	0

Illustrative Case

A 41-year-old woman presented to us with a 15-year history of occipital headache and 1-year history of decreased hearing. Neurological examination was positive for absent nerve VIII function on the left. CT scans showed an enhancing tumor involving the left pyramid and the left temporo-occipital bone (Fig. 17.1 a, b). With the patient in the supine position, head tilted to the right, a lateral left suboccipital craniectomy was extended over the temporal region in preparation for a supra-infratentorial approach. The temporo-occipital bone was hyperostotic and diffusely infiltrated by tumor and was removed with clean margins exposing completely the transverse and sigmoid sinus and the posterior temporal dura. A mastoidectomy and partial petrosectomy including the labyrinth were then performed with exposure and preservation of nerve VII in the fallopian canal. The sigmoid sinus and the adjacent involved dura were then removed, and the intradural, supra- and infratentorial tumor was completely removed. The dura was grafted with lyophilized dura and the bone defect reconstructed with acrylic, a subgaleal drain inserted, and the scalp closed as usual. The postoperative course was uneventful, and the patient was discharged with an remarkable neurological examination with the exception of the left-sided deafness already present preoperatively. Postoperative CT scan is shown in Fig. 17.1

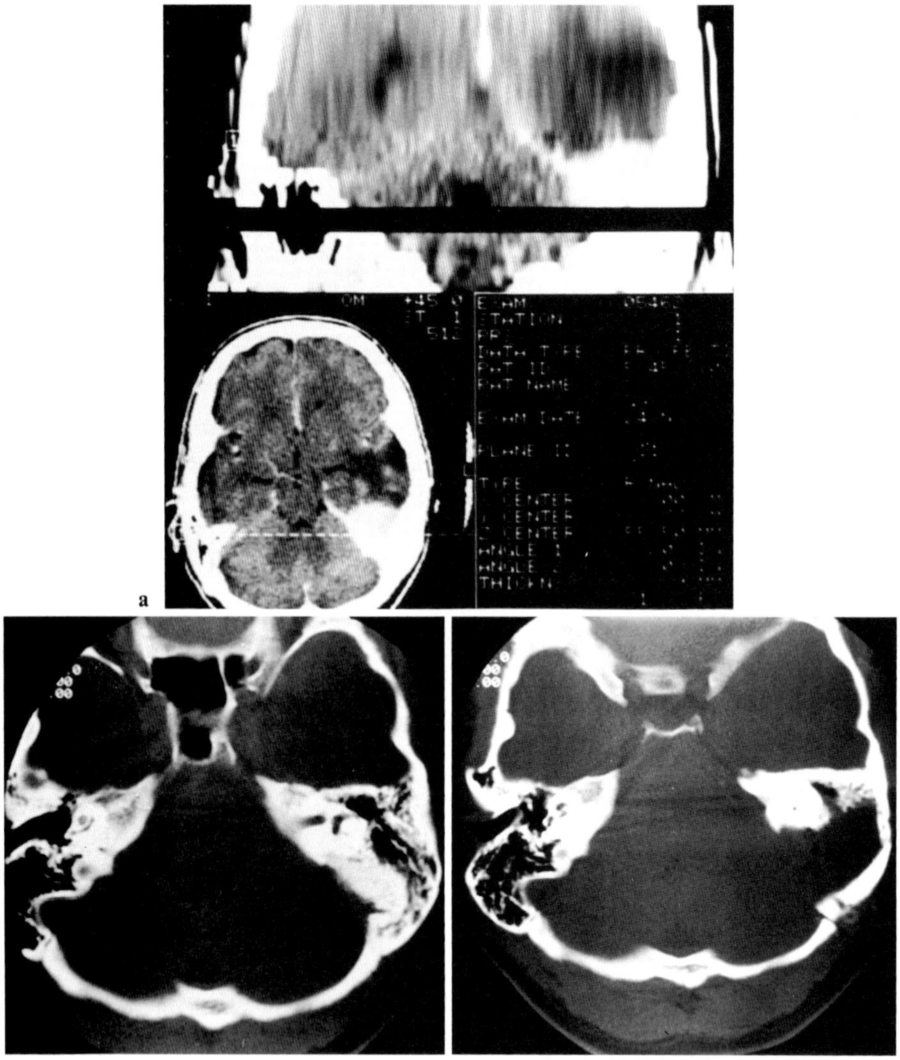

Fig. 17.1 a – c. A 41-year-old woman with meningioma of the petrous pyramid and of the temporo-occipital bone. **a** Preoperative CT scan shows the tumor in the middle and posterior cranial fossae. **b** CT scan obtained with bony window shows the extensive pyramidal involvement. **c** Postoperative CT scan shows the extent of bone removal

CHAPTER 18

Intraosseous Meningiomas

General Considerations

Meningiomas limited primarily to the bone (intraosseous or intradiploic meningiomas) are rarely seen [8, 17]. Since the term meningioma was introduced and popularized by Cushing in 1922 [4] there have been sporadic reports of intraosseous meningiomas involving the temporal bone [2, 6, 9, 11, 12], bony orbit [5, 7, 14, 15, 18], and other areas of the skull [1, 10, 13, 16, 18]. These tumors are extremely rare, but no age group is spared – a case was reported in a 7-month-old child [3]. The frequency of intraosseous meningiomas is not known exactly. Cushing in his classic monograph of meningiomas did not mention any such case [4], and the frequency of primary intraosseous meningiomas has not been reported in any major neurosurgical series. In the course of their growth intraosseous meningiomas may eventually thin out and break through the bone (just as subdural meningiomas invade bone by breaking through the dura), adding an extraosseous portion to their mainly intraosseous tumor, and may eventually infiltrate the dura locally. Their primary intraosseous origin may be inferred from the location of the main tumor mass and from the very limited dural invasion [1, 18].

Personal Series

We have seen four cases of primary intraosseous meningiomas, accounting for 1.8% of skull base meningiomas ($n = 217$) and 1% of intracranial meningiomas ($n = 383$); it is interesting that all our cases originated in the skull base. Table 18.1 summarizes our material. These four patients are described in detail below (see "Illustrative Cases").

Illustrative Cases

Case 1. A 21-year-old man had been complaining of left-sided facial weakness for the past 9 years. Neurological examination was positive for left peripheral facial palsy. CT scans showed a lesion in the medial anterior portion of the left pyramid with a soft tissue density component (Fig. 18.1 a, b). MRI confirmed the CT findings (Fig. 18.1 c). EMG demonstrated complete denervation of the muscles innervated by the left facial nerve. At surgery, via a posterior subtemporal approach, an intraosseous tumor involving the medial anterior portion of the left pyramid and extending into the middle ear was removed, together with a small extradural-extraosseous portion of the tumor abuting on the basal temporal dura that was also resected. Postoperatively the patient was deaf. Pathology showed a meningioma. Postoperative CT scans showed no evidence of the tumor (Fig. 18.1 d, e). The complete facial palsy was treated 8 months later with a temporal muscle transfer. The patient remains disease-free 13 months postoperatively.

Table 18.1. Intraosseous meningiomas

Number	4
Age: range/mean/median (years)	21 – 66/48/52
Women/men	2/2
Symptom (most common)	See text
Sign (most common)	See text
Tumor removal	
Total	4
Subtotal	0
Outcome	
Good	4
Fair	0
Poor	0
Deaths	0

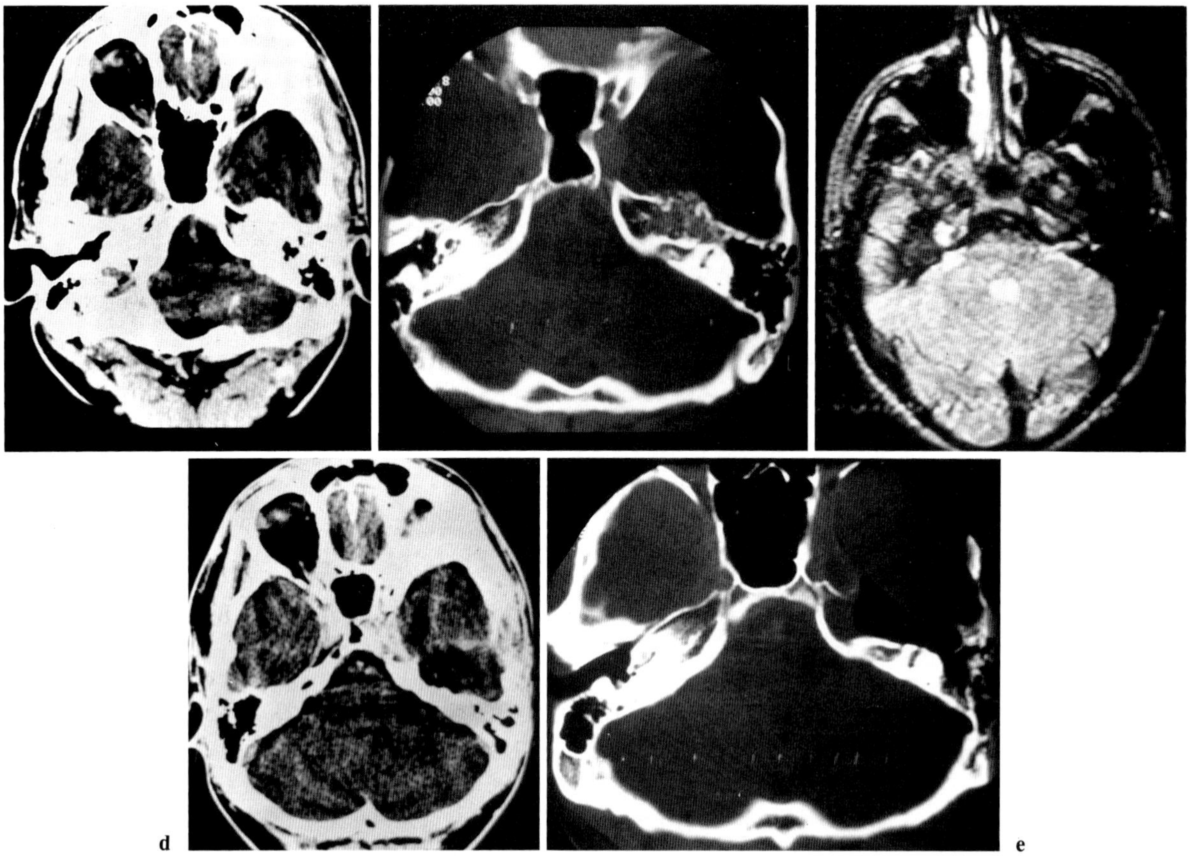

18.1 a b, c

d e

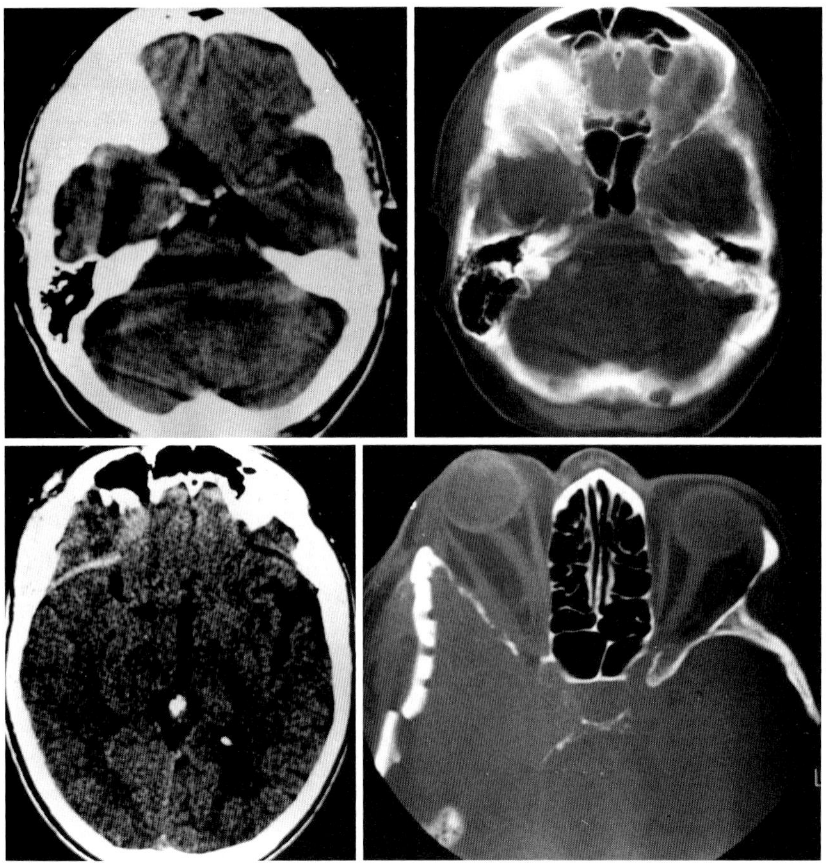

18.2 a b

c d

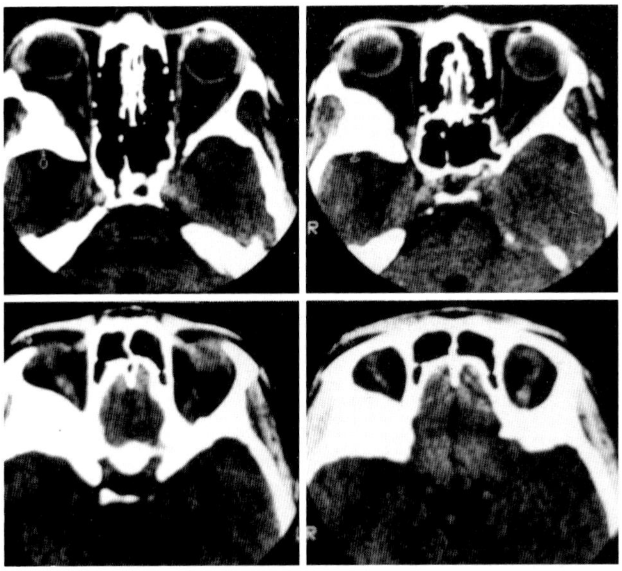

18.3 a

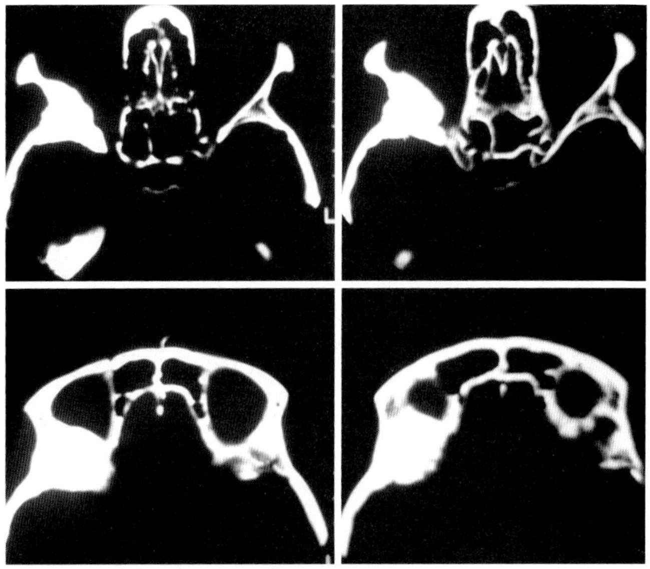

b

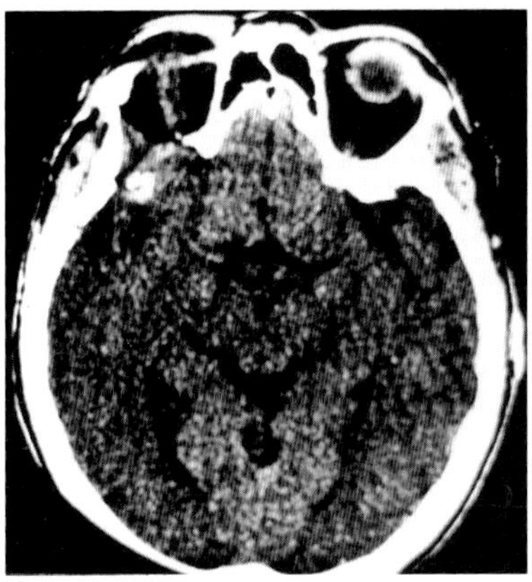

c

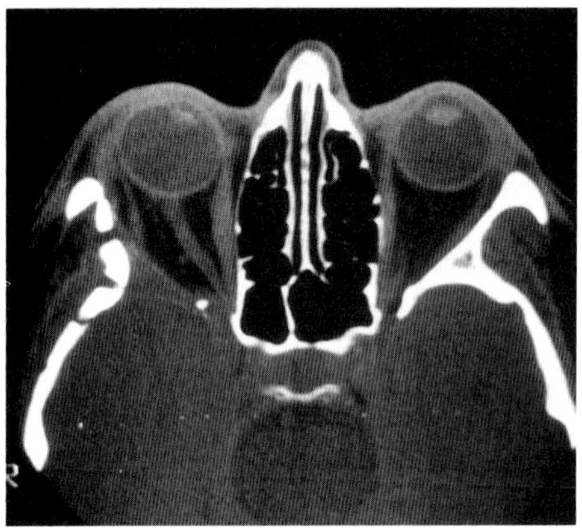

d

Fig. 18.1 a–e. A 21-year-old man with left complete peripheral facial palsy and intrapetrous meningioma. **a** CT scan shows a bony lesion in the anterior aspect of the left pyramid. **b** A soft tissue density mass protruding in the middle fossa from the anterior pyramid is well demonstrated in this CT scan with bone window. **c** MRI scan, T2 weighted, shows an hyperintense lesion in the left pyramid. **d, e** Postoperative CT scans show complete tumor removal. The tumor cavity is best appreciated using bone window (**e**)

Fig. 18.3 a–d. A 55-year-old woman with painful right-sided exophthalmos. **a, b** CT scans without (**a**) and with (**b**) bone window show a hyperostotic tumor involving the greater and lesser wings of the sphenoid on the right side. **c, d** Postoperative CT scans show complete tumor removal. The acrylic cranioplastic is well seen using bone window (**d**)

Fig. 18.2 a–d. A 66-year-old woman with right-sided exophthalmos. **a, b** CT scans show a hyperostotic tumor of the lateral and superior orbital wall. **c, d** Postoperative CT scans demonstrate no evidence of tumor. The extent of the bony removal and the acrylic cranioplastic are well seen using bone window (**d**)

Case 2. A 66-year-old woman was seen by us because of progressive protrusion of the right eye of 10 years' duration. Neurological examination yielded normal results, and physical examination showed a 4-mm exophthalmos on the right. CT scans showed a hyperostotic tumor involving the lateral and superior orbital wall on the right side (Fig. 18.2 a, b). A frontotemporal craniotomy was performed, and an intraosseous tumor involving the orbital roof without invasion of the orbital cavity or of the frontotemporal dura was completely removed. Acrylic was used to reconstruct the bony defect. Pathology showed a meningioma. The postoperative course was uneventful, and the patient was discharged neurologically intact. Postoperative CT scans showed complete tumor removal (Fig. 18.2 c, d).

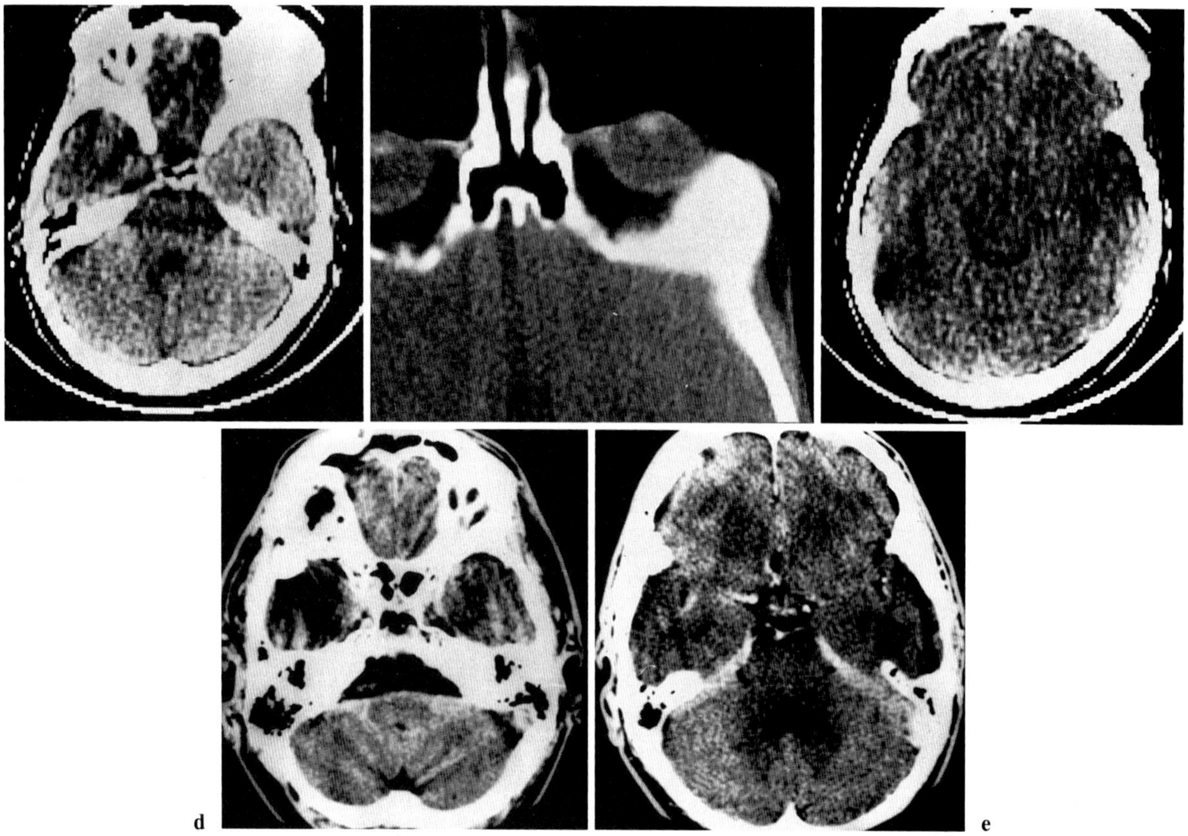

a, b c d e

Case 3. A 55-year-old woman complained of pain and protrusion of the right eye as well as of occasional double vision when looking to the left; this had been present for the past 3 years. Results on neurological examination was negative. Physical examination showed a 2-mm right-sided exophthalmos and swelling of the right upper eyelid. CT scans showed an intraosseous tumor involving the lateral and superior wall of the orbit and the anterior portion of the temporal squama on the right (Fig. 18.3 a, b). Via a frontotemporal craniotomy an intraosseous tumor involving the greater and lesser wings of the sphenoid in correspondence of the lateral and superior orbital wall and of the anterior part of the temporal squama was completely removed. The frontotemporal dura and orbital cavity were free of tumor. The bony defect was repaired using acrylic. Pathological examination showed a meningioma. Postoperative course was uncomplicated, and postoperative CT scans showed no evidence of residual tumor (Fig. 18.3 c, d).

Fig. 18.4 a – e. A 49-year-old man with right-sided ocular pain. **a – c** CT scans demonstrate an hyperostotic tumor of the lower frontal and of the sphenoid bone. **d, e** CT scans, 8 years after the operation, show no evidence of tumor

Case 4. A 49-year-old man sought medical attention because of pain in the right eye and right lower forehead for the past 6 years. Neurological examination yielded negative results. CT scans showed an intraosseous tumor involving the lateral and superior orbital wall and the right lower frontal bone in correspondence of the frontal sinus (Fig. 18.4 a – c). Via a right frontotemporal craniotomy an intraosseous tumor involving the right frontal sinus, the greater and lesser wings of the sphenoid at the level of the lateral, the superior orbital wall, and the temporal squama was totally removed. The skull was reconstructed using acrylic. Pathological examination showed a meningioma. Postoperative course was uneventful. Control CT scans, 8 years after the operation, showed no tumor recurrence (Fig. 18.4 d, e).

References

1. Azar-Kia B, Sarwar M, Allan Marc J, Schechter MM (1974) Intraosseous meningioma. Neuroradiology 6:246–253
2. Buehrle R, Goodman WS, Wortzman G (1972) Meningioma of the temporal bone. Can J Otolaryngol 1:16–20
3. Choux M, Gomiez A, Choux R, Vigouroux RP (1975) Diagnostic and therapeutic problems concerning tumors of the vault. Childs Brain 1:207–216
4. Cushing H, Eisenhardt L (1962) Meningiomas, their classification, regional behaviour, life history, and surgical end results, 2nd edn. Hafner, New York
5. Dahlmann J (1951) Osteoblastisches Meningiom im Orbitaldach. Fortschr Geb Röntgenstr 74:306–315
6. Guzowski J, Paparella M, Nageswara K, Hoshion T (1986) Meningiomas of the temporal bone. Laryngoscope 86:1141–1146
7. Kobayashi S, Kyoshima K, Nakagawa F, Sugita K, Maruyama Y (1980) Diploic meningioma of the orbital roof. Surg Neurol 13:277–281
8. Lee W, Tu Y, Liu M (1988) Primary intraosseous malignant meningioma of the skull. Case report. Neurosurgery 23:505–508
9. Maniglia AJ (1978) Intra- and extracranial meningiomas involving the temporal bone. Laryngoscope [Suppl] 12
10. McWhorter JM, Ghatak NR, Kelly DL (1976) Extracranial meningioma presenting as lytic skull lesion. Surg Neurol 5:223–224
11. Nager GT (1964) Meningiomas involving the temporal bone; clinical and clinicopathological aspects. Thomas, Springfield
12. Parisier SC, Som PM, Shugar JMA, Marovitz WF (1978) The evaluation of middle ear meningiomas using computerized axial tomography. Laryngoscope 88: 1170–1177
13. Pendergrass EP, Hope JW (1953) An extracranial meningioma with no apparent intracranial source. A J R 70:967–970
14. Pompili A, Caroli F, Cattani F, Iachetti M (1983) Intradiploic meningioma of the orbital roof. Neurosurgery 12:565–568
15. Reale F, Delfini R, Cintorino A (1978) An intradiploic meningioma of the orbital roof. Case report. Ophthalmologica 177:82–87
16. Siegel GT, Anderson PJ (1966) Extracalvarial meningioma. Case report. J Neurosurg 25:83–86
17. Voorhies RM, Sundaresan N (1985) Tumors of the skull. In: Wilkins RH, Rengachary SS (eds) Neurosurgery, vol 1. McGraw-Hill, New York, pp 984–1001
18. Wagman AD, Weiss EK, Riggs HE (1960) Hyperplasia of the skull associated with intraosseous meningioma in the absence of gross tumor. J Neuropathol Exp Neurol 19:111–115

CHAPTER 19

Pathobiology and Neuropathology of Meningiomas

G. F. WALTER

Pathobiology

Histogenesis

The meninges include the dura mater, the arachnoidal cap cells and granulations, the subarachnoidal blood vessels and fibroblasts, and the pia. The changing composition of these histological elements is responsible for the different subtypes of meningiomas. Intraventricular meningiomas arise from the tela choroidea of the choroid plexus, hemangiopericytic meningiomas from mesenchymal perivascular cells or, in a different view, from meningothelial cells transformed into pericytes. Thus, meningiomas are tumors with both neuroectodermal and mesenchymal histogenesis [40, 101].

Incidences

Meningiomas represent about 15% of all primary intracranial tumors. This means about 1.3 meningiomas per 100 000 persons per year, given an incidence of 8.2 primary intracranial tumors per year [39, 94, 102]. Female patients predominate, with 60%–65% in benign meningiomas, whereas no sexual prevalence can be found in malignant variants. Symptomatic meningiomas are most commonly detected in the middle decades of life, with a peak of incidence between the fifth and sixth decades. Intraventricular meningiomas have an incidence of about 2% among all meningiomas [17] and account for about 10%–15% of all intraventricular tumors [38, 103]. The occurrence of intracranial meningiomas in infancy is extremely rare [80], in childhood still very rare with about 1.5% of all primary intracranial tumors [58]. In contrast to adults, intraventricular meningiomas in children have an incidence of about 15% among all meningiomas [60]. Intracranial meningiomas found incidentally at autopsy include about 2% of all autopsy cases [74]. The prevalence increases with age. There is a male-to-female ratio of approximately 1 : 3 in all age groups [66], whereas a previous study [97] showed no sex dominance. In 231 cases reported by Nakasu et al. [66], the necropsy incidence increased with age, for instance from 1.2% in the fifth decade of life to 4.6% in the ninth decade (2.3% of the total of 10 033 autopsies). Multiple tumors comprised 8.2% in (two to four meningiomas) patients without stigmata of neurofibromatosis or diffuse meningiomatosis. Aging seems to be an important factor in multiplicity.

Spinal meningiomas constitute approximately 25% of all spinal canal tumors [67]. There is also a marked preponderance of about 80% among elderly women.

Molecular Biology

Recent advances in cytogenetics have provided new insights into the mechanisms responsible for the development of meningiomas. The loss of regions on the long arm of chromosome 22, possibly containing a tumor suppressor gene that is important in the growth control of cells deriving from the neural crest, has been found not only in meningiomas but also in schwannomas, neurofibromas, type II neurofibromatosis (bilateral acoustic neurinomatosis), and astrocytomas.

Cytogenetical studies have shown that meningioma karyotypes are frequently characterized by a loss of one of the chromosome 22 homologues. Although some abnormalities such as loss or deletion have been observed on other chromosomes, these were far less consistent than those on chromosome

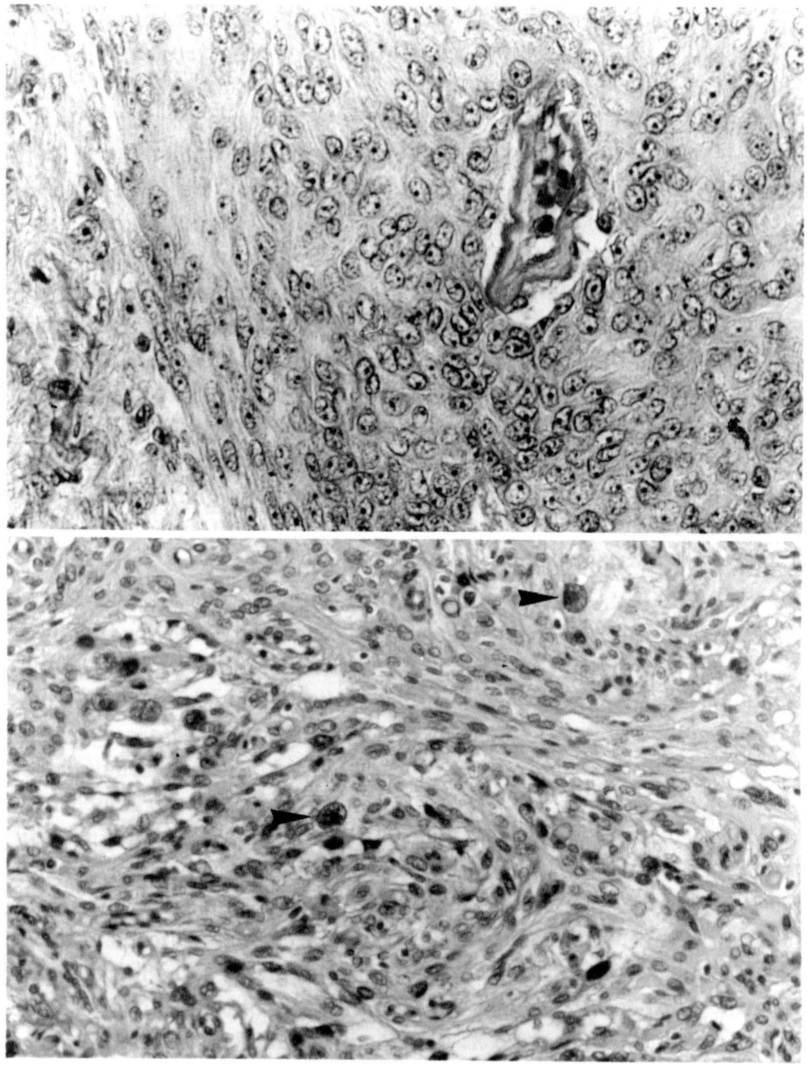

Fig. 19.1. **a** Meningotheliomatous meningioma with syncytial appearance and characteristic pale nuclei (Masson trichrome, ×170). **b** Cellular polymorphism with giant nuclei (*arrowheads*; HE, ×100)

whorls, often around capillaries and possibly with central psammoma bodies. Meningothelial and fibrous areas are mixed.

Psammomatous meningiomas (Fig. 19.2c) contain large amounts of calcified psammoma bodies and preferentially occur along the spinal cord in aged women [32].

Angiomatous meningiomas (Fig. 19.3) exhibit many large and small blood vessels, often with a marked fibrous hyaline thickening of the vessel wall. The intervening tissue may be meningothelial or fibrous.

Hemangioblastic meningiomas (Fig. 19.4) are composed of capillaries that are separated by lipid-containing stromal cells with clear cytoplasm. They

Fig. 19.2. **a** Fibrous meningioma with elongated cell strands (Masson trichrome, ×20). **b** Transitional meningioma with typical whorls (Masson trichrome, ×170). **c** Psammomatous meningioma with calcified psammoma bodies (Masson trichrome, ×60)

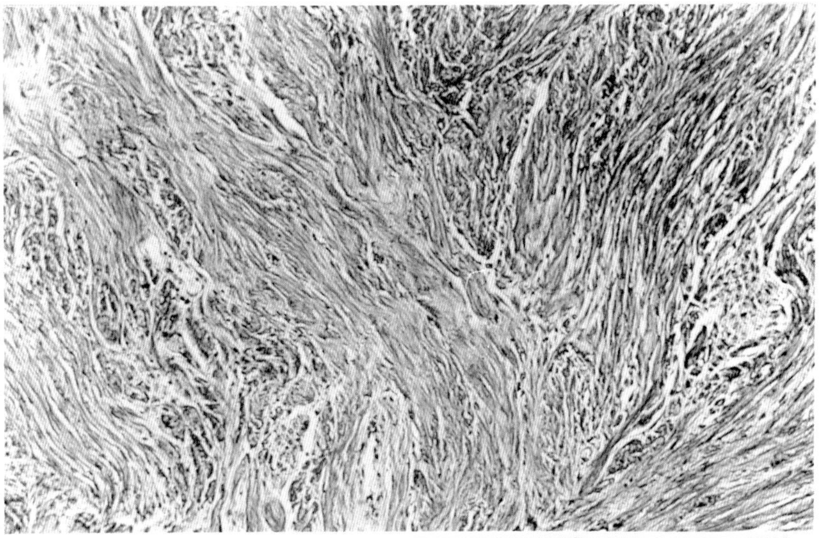

a

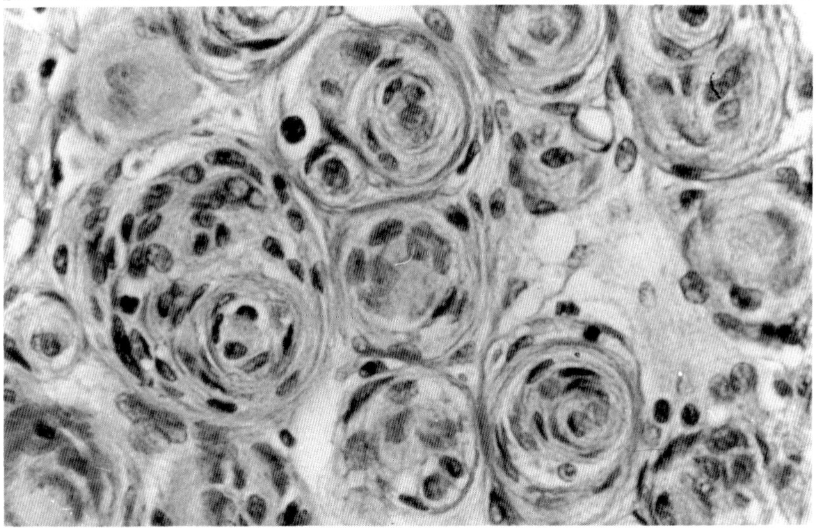

b

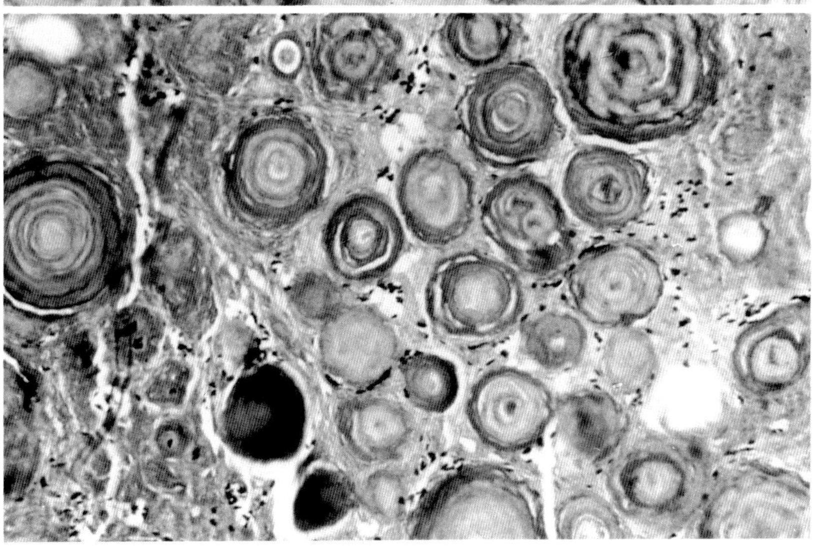

c

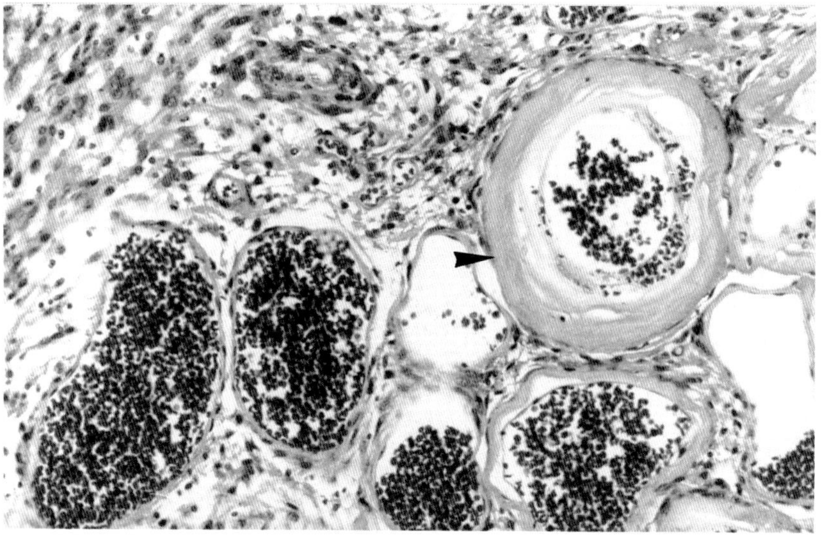

19.3

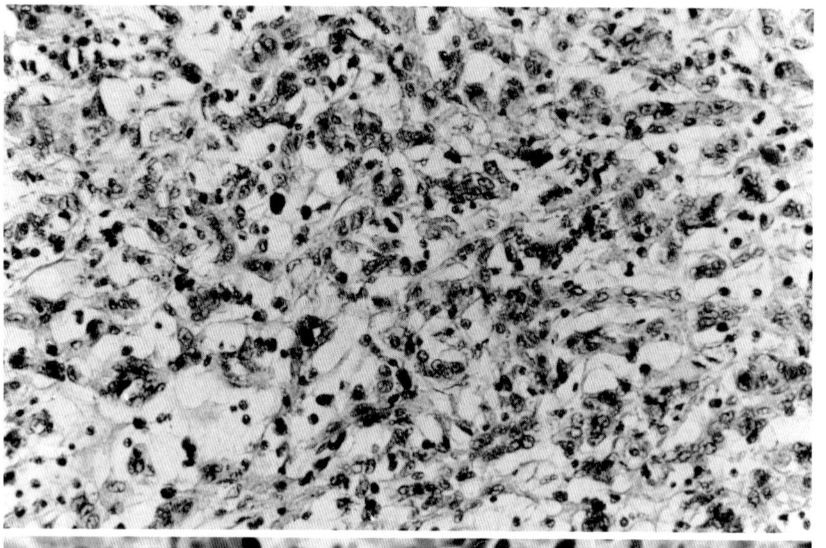

19.4 a

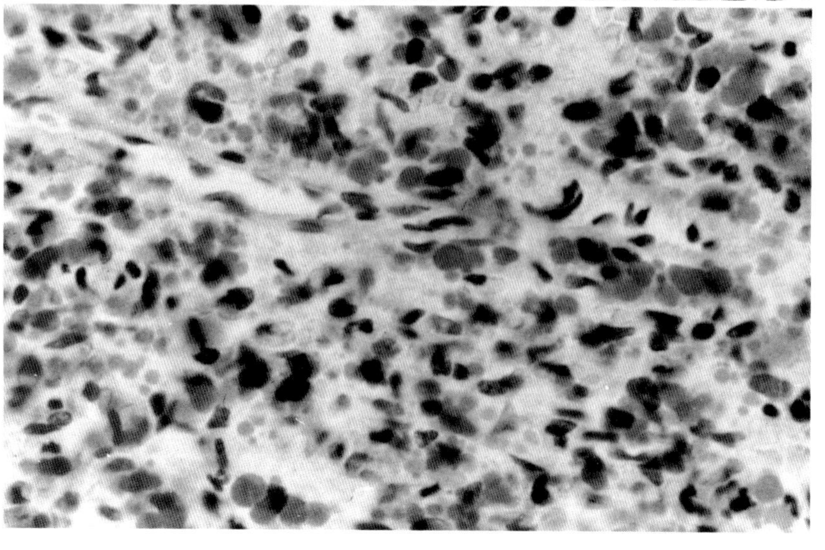

b

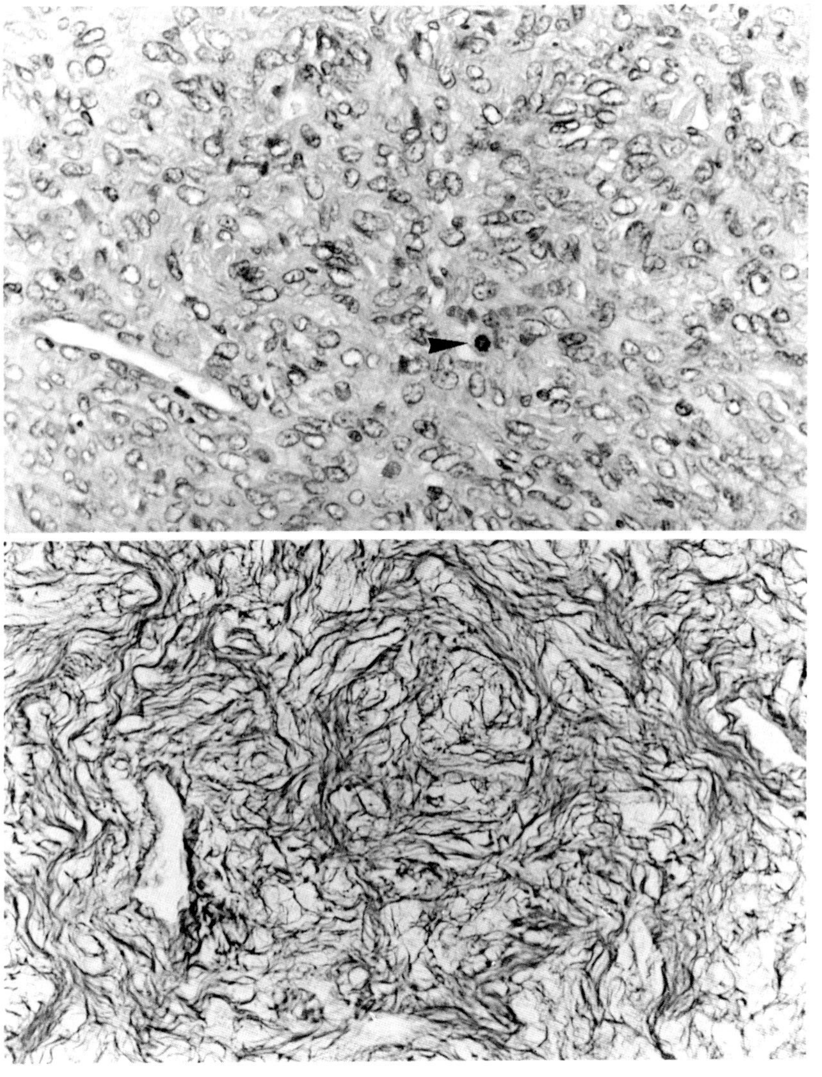

Fig. 19.5 a Hemangiopericytic meningioma with densely packed cells and a mitosis (*arrowhead*; HE, ×170). **b** Hemangiopericytic meningioma with demonstration of the abundant perivascular reticulin (Gomori silver impregnation, ×100)

Fig. 19.3. Angiomatous meningioma with many blood vessels, some exhibiting a hyaline thickening of the vessel wall (*arrowhead*; Masson trichrome, ×100)

Fig. 19.4. a Hemangioblastic meningioma with clear stromal cells (Masson trichrome, ×100). **b** Hemangioblastic meningioma with demonstration of the lipid droplets (*light grey*) within the stromal cells (oil red 0, ×170)

may be regarded as hemangioblastoma of the meninges, being histologically indistinguishable from the hemangioblastoma of the cerebellum (Lindau tumor).

Hemangiopericytic meningiomas (Fig. 19.5) consist of capillaries surrounded by densely packed cells with little, insufficiently separated cytoplasm. The nuclei are often pale, resembling the nuclei of meningothelial tissue, but chromatin-rich nuclei may also be found. Mitoses are frequent. There are no whorls or psammoma bodies. Pericellular and perivascular reticulin is abundant. They may be regarded as hemangiopericytomas of the meninges and are histologically indistinguishable from hemangiopericytomas elsewhere in the body. Metastases are possible.

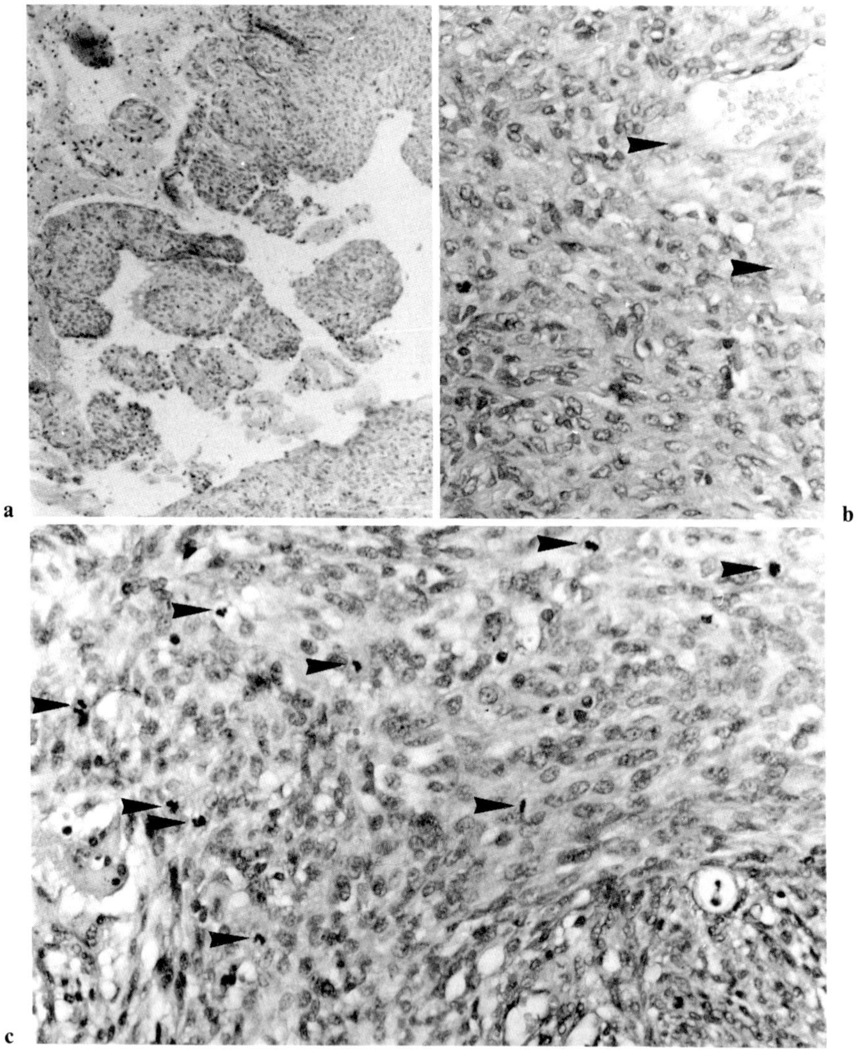

Fig. 19.6. **a** Papillary meningioma, overview over the papillary pattern (HE, ×20). **b** Anaplastic meningioma with necrosis (*arrowheads*; HE, ×100). **c** Anaplastic meningioma with high rate of mitoses (*arrowheads*; HE, ×100)

Papillary meningiomas (Fig. 19.6a) may have an epithelial cell morphology within the papillary formations themselves. The papillary pattern is often associated with histological features indicative of malignancy such as many mitoses. In fact, the papillary pattern may be pseudopapillary in the form of vital, remaining tissue rests around stromal blood vessels in a largely necrotic tumor. In my opinion, the papillary meningioma should therefore not be regarded as a separate subtype but rather as a special growth pattern of an anaplastic meningiomas. As in other anaplastic meningiomas, metastases are possible.

Anaplastic meningiomas (Fig. 19.6b, c) are meningiomas belonging to one or another subtype which display – possibly only focally – signs of anaplasia such as aggressive local invasiveness, infiltration of the underlying brain, poor differentiation, a high mitotic rate with typical and atypical mitoses, and necrosis. A rapid rate of recurrence and remote metastases are possible. They are not to be confused with primary undifferentiated meningeal sarcomas, e.g., a fibrosarcoma.

In rare metaplastic variants, pluripotential mesenchymal stem cells may undergo a metaplastic differentiation into fat cells, bone, or cartilage causing tumors called lipoblastic, osteoblastic, or

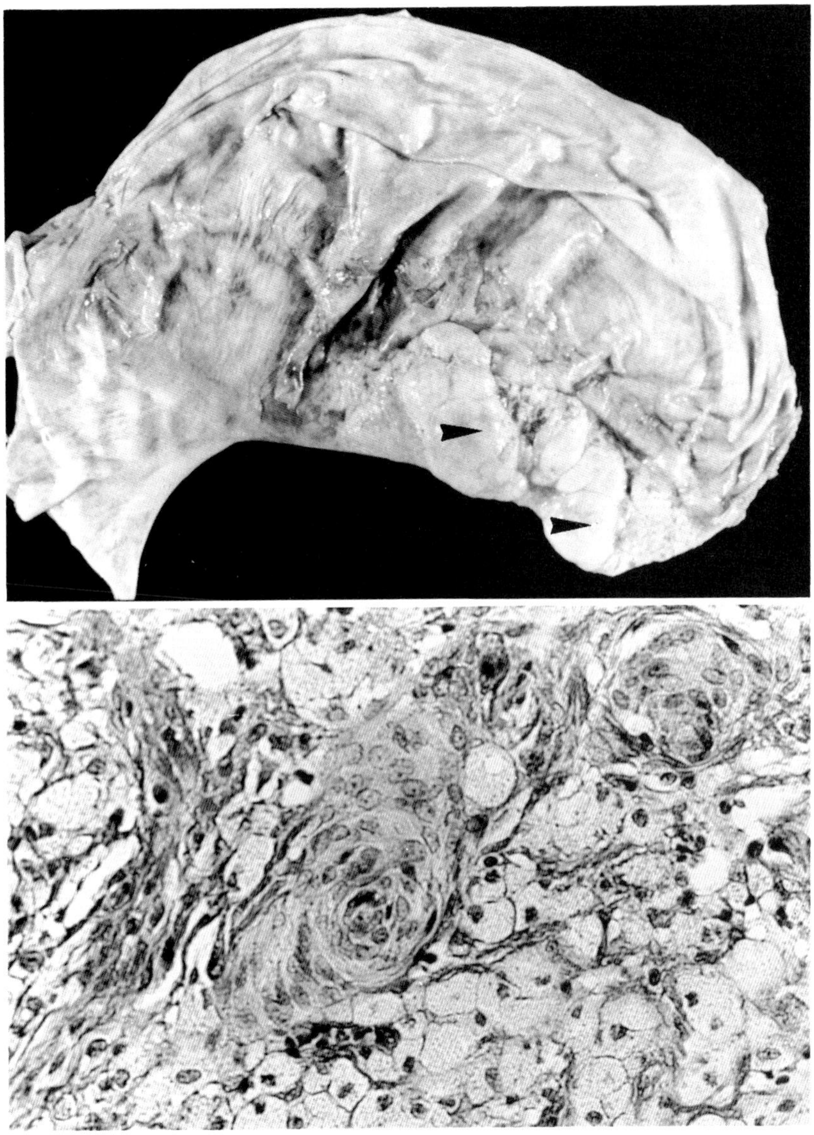

a

b

chondroblastic meningiomas. A mesenchymal storage phenomenon is shown by the exanthomatous meningioma (Fig. 19.7), with large portions of the tumor consisting of meningothelial cells transformed in xanthomatous foam cells.

Cystic meningiomas appear in the form of macrocystic or microcystic tumors. Macrocystic meningiomas can be classified in different types according to the site of the cavity and the relationship that it has with the tumor and surrounding parenchyma (reviewed in [22]). Microcystic meningiomas (Fig. 19.8a) are characterized by a diffuse vacuolation and a rich vascular network with hyalin change and increased numbers of mast cells [79, 82]. The microcystic alterations are associated with local vascular permeability disturbances. A microcystic variant described as myxomatous meningioma is characterized by myxoid degenerations and a high recurrency rate [20, 28, 82]. The myxomatous cystic changes may perhaps be regarded as evidence for a mucoid secretion of the tumor cells, but chondromyxoid changes may also be supposed. Masson's so-called humid form (*forme humide*) of

Fig. 19.7. a Xanthomatous meningioma of the falx with golden-yellow macroscopic appearance (*arrowheads*). **b** Xanthomatous meningioma with a typical whorl and surrounding foam cells (Masson trichrome, ×170)

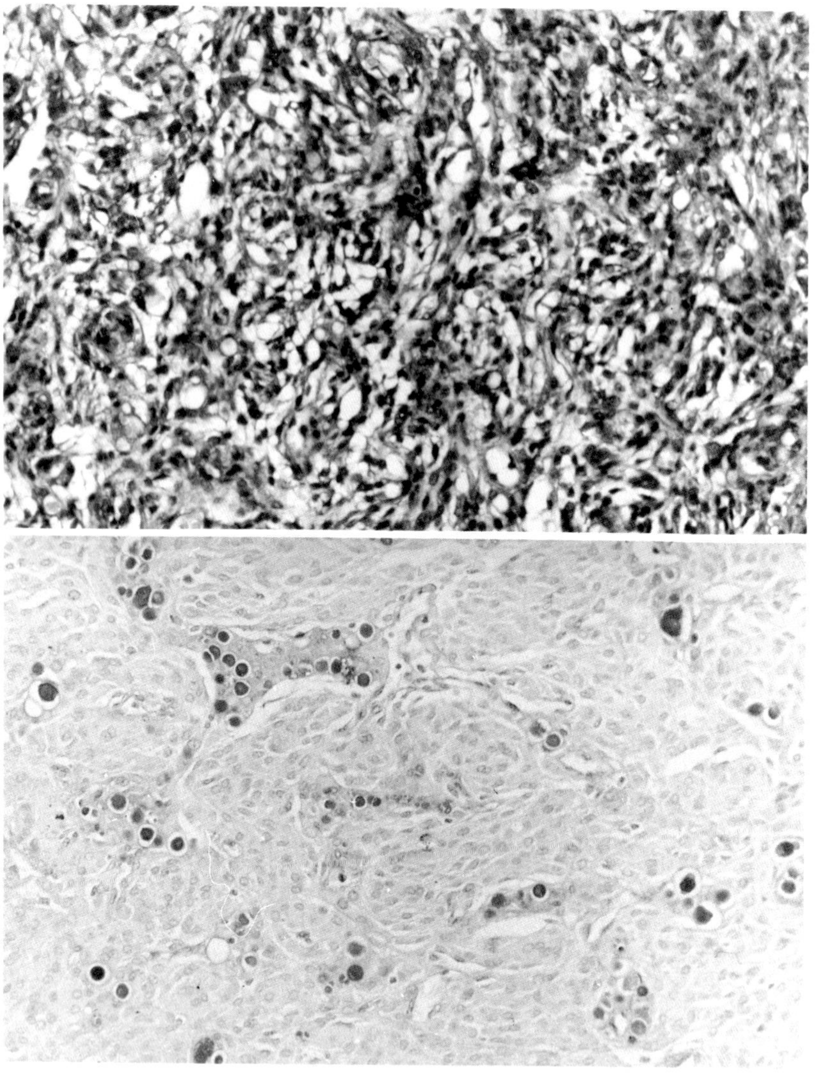

a

b

Fig. 19.8. **a** Microcystic meningioma with diffuse vacuolation (HE, ×100). **b** Secretory meningioma with pseudopsammoma bodies (PAS, ×100)

meningiomas represents a tumor that has undergone both mucoid and lipid degeneration, resulting in a bubbly, watery, "humid" macroscopic aspect.

Another secondary change in certain benign meningiomas, in the form of PAS-positive hyaline inclusions or pseudopsammoma bodies (Fig. 19.8b) which are not calcified, has also been ascribed to a secretory activity of the tumor cells, because ultrastructural studies have revealed intracellular ductules lines by microvilli around the hyaline inclusions. Alguacil-Garcia et al. [4] discuss secretory meningioma even as a distinct subtype, which from my point of view is justified.

Other meningeal tumors such as meningeal sarcomas, xanthomatous tumors, and primary melanotic tumors show no signs of having arisen from a preexisting meningioma and are not taken into consideration in the present description.

Ultrastructure. The ultrastructure of the mesothelium-like arachnoidal cap cells and the leptomeningeal and pachymeningeal connective tissue was comprehensively investigated first by Andres [5]. The electron microscopic features of normal meningothelial elements are identical to the findings in meningiomas of all subtypes but the hemangiopericytic one. They show complex cytoplasmic interdigitations separated by parallel-running membranes. Adjacent membranes are bound with desmosomes. In some cells, intracytoplasmic intermediate filaments of the cytoskeleton may be seen, especially in the elongated cells of the fibrous subtype. Fibrous subtypes have also a considerable participation of interstitial collagen filaments.

A principal ultrastructural difference is exhibited by the cells of the hemangiopericytic subtype. They show blunt cytoplasmic edges and often contain abundant intermediate filaments as well as microfilaments forming dense bodies. Interstitial basement membranes presumably represent the intercellular reticulin fiber network demonstrable by light microscopy [78]. There are neither cytoplasmic interdigitations nor desmosomes in this subtype.

Immunhistochemistry. Immunohistochemical methods seem to be appropriate tools to obtain answers as to the true histogenetic derivation of the various subtypes of meningiomas. In meningiomas, intermediate filament proteins and some other antigens can be used for the immunohistochemical characterization of the tumor (Table 19.2).

The cytoskeleton consists of different types of intracytoplasmic filamentous structures. Besides microfilaments (5–7 nm) and microtubules (22 nm), intermediate-sized filaments measuring 8–11 nm are common in almost all eukaryotic cells. These intermediate filaments are a multigene family of related polypeptides comprising five classes: cytokeratins, the neurofilament triplet, glial fibrillary acidic protein (GFAP), desmin, and vimentin. Vimentin is the major intermediate filament in meningiomas and has also been demonstrated in normal arachnoidal cap cells [84]. The presence of cytokeratin filaments which are characteristic for epithelial cells was more controversal. However, several studies have confirmed that cytokeratins can be found at least in some meningiomas [59, 64, 92, 99]. Cells do not usually contain more than one intermediate filament type, but when they do – for instance, during embryonic development – one of the two types is always vimentin [69]. As in meningiomas, a coexpression of vimentin and cytokeratins can also be found in mesotheliomas [15, 46], an indication that mesothelium and meninges may occupy a kind of intermediate position between mesenchymal and epithelial tissue.

Table 19.2. Immunohistochemistry of meningiomas

	"Typical" meningioma	Hemangiopericytic meningioma
Cytokeratins	+ or –	–
Neurofilament	–	–
GFAP	–	–
Desmin	–	+
Vimentin	+	+
Desmoplakin	+	–
Factor VIII	–	+
Laminin	+ or –	+

Desmoplakins were originally identified as protein components of desmosomal plaques present in epithelial cells, but they can also be shown in the desmosomes of meningothelial tissue. The association of desmosomes with vimentin filaments is unique for arachnoidal cells so that positive immunohistochemical stainings of desmoplakin and vimentin are characteristic for all subtypes of meingiomas with the exception of the hemangiopericytic [84]. Factor VIII-related antigen can be used as specific marker for normal and neoplastic endothelium and laminin as a marker for basement membranes. Laminin is a major glycoprotein component of basement membranes.

The immunohistochemical results in hemangiopercytic meningiomas are still very controversial; therefore, the staining reactions listed in Table 19.2 represent results in only the majority of tumors. Hemangiopericytic meningiomas and extracranial soft tissue hemangiopericytomas show a negative immunoreactivity for epithelial membrane antigen (EMA) whereas all other subtypes react positively for EMA [35, 62]. Kawano et al. [37] report positive staining for vimentin and desmin in cell cultures of hemangiopericytic subtypes, suggesting that they have something in common with vascular fibroblasts and muscle cells. These results and ultrastructural investigations [65] support the concept that hemangiopericytic meningiomas originate from vascular but not from meningothelial tissue. On the other hand, Holden et al. [31] report that arachnoidal granulations and all subtypes of meningiomas including the hemangiopericytic gave a positive staining for vimentin and a variably positive staining for cytokeratins, whereas normal pericytes and soft tissue hemangiopericytomas were negative for both vimentin and cytokeratins. They concluded that the hemangiopericytic meningioma is a variant of meningioma and is not of pericytic origin. However, according to my experience, the histological recognition of the hemangiopericytic subtype of meningioma normally poses no problems, so that the cytological derivation remains an academic question.

Lectin Histochemistry. The cell surface is covered by sugar chains or oligosaccharides which are important in cell-cell recognition. These carbohydrates react with lectins, sugar-binding proteins, or glycoproteins which originate from plants or animals. Lectins agglutinate cells and precipitate glycoproteins. The value of lectins lies in their ability to identify minor differences among the carbohydrates.

Ulex europaeus type I lectin, an even more sensitive marker for endothelial cells than factor VIII, was used for studying vascular meningiomas [95]. An extensive study of different patterns of lectin binding in meningiomas using 11 different lectins was carried out by Kleinert and Radner [42]. *Ulex europaeus* (gorse) type I agglutinin, *Triticum vulgare* (wheatgerm) agglutinin, and *Helix pomatia* (snail) agglutinin bind to endothelial cells. *Glycine max* (soybean) agglutinin and *Bauhinia purpurea alba* (orchard tree) agglutinin, in a granular fashion, bind to fibrous areas. *Vicia fava* (vetch) agglutinin and *Concanavalia ensiformis* (jack bean) agglutinin bind to meningothelial areas. *Arachis hypogaea* (peanut) agglutinin and *Laburnum alpinum* (laburnum) agglutinin bind to meningothelial and fibrous areas. *Dolichos biflorus* (horse gram) agglutinin and *Limax flavus* (slug) agglutinin give no reaction.

Grading

The WHO classification uses a four-grade scale to signify the biological behavior and the prognosis of intracranial tumors. Grade I is considered benign, and grades II (semibenign), III (relatively malignant), and IV (highly malignant) indicate increasing degrees of malignancy.

Meningiomas of the subtypes 1–6 (Table 19.1) as well as the rare metaplastic variants correspond histologically to grade I. The hemangiopericytic subtype tends to be more aggressive, with more rapid recurrence and invasive growth. It corresponds histologically to grade II. The papillary subtype and all kinds of anaplastic meningiomas correspond histologically to grade III.

Borges [11] found that immunostaining meningiomas for laminin may be predictive of biological behavior. In a study of 50 meningiomas, he noted that the tumors which were histologically benign demonstrated intact basement membrane staining. Anaplastic meningiomas lacked any immunostaining except around some blood vessels.

It is not uncommon to find perivascular or diffusely scattered foci of lymphocytes or plasma cells, or both, as well as histiocytes in meningiomas [7], which on occasion may cause diagnostic difficulties. Investigations of the cellular immune response have shown that the numbers of macrophages and T and CD8 lymphocytes in meningiomas seem to be related to atypical histological features. The presence of these cells raises questions concerning the host's immune response and the possible relationship of this to prognosis [76].

Cell Kinetics. The cell cycle proceeds in phases. After a mitosis (M phase), the interphase (I phase) starts, which can be divided into a variably long lasting stable gap (G_1 phase) followed by the synthesis (S phase) and replication of DNA, which is again followed by a stable gap (G_2 phase) of relatively constant duration before the next M phase begins. In a more correct way than counting the mitosis rate for grading of meningiomas, studies of cell kinetics calculates the ratio of proliferating to nonproliferating tumor cells. Cell kinetics can be measured with ^{67}Ki antibody or anti-bromodeoxyuridine (anti-BrdU) antibody. ^{67}Ki is known to react with an antigen that is present in the nuclei only of proliferating cells (S, G_2, and M phases)(and is absent in the G_1 phase of the cell cycle [12]. Immunostaining of proliferating cells with ^{67}Ki antibody provides a reliable means of estimating the growth fractions of normal and neoplastic cell populations. In well-differentiated meningiomas, 0.2% – 1.6% ^{67}Ki positive cells can be counted [12, 54]. To my knowledge, there are no results for anaplastic meningiomas. Another possibility is the use of intravenously administered BrdU, a thymidine analogue which is incorporated into nuclear DNA during the S phase. Using an anti-BrdU monoclonal antibody for immunohistochemical investigations in the resected meningioma, a labeling index can be obtained by counting the ratio of BrdU-positive nuclei to all nuclei. The labeling indices of benign meningiomas are usually less than 1%. In anaplastic meningiomas, labeling indices vary between 3% and 9% [13, 34, 98]. As BrdU-labeling indices correlate with the tumor doubling time, as estimated from serial computed tomography, they may be used for the prediction of tumor growth [13]. An important disadvantage of the BrdU uptake method must be mentioned. The potentially carcinogenic BrdU must be administered to the patient, and with this method the size of the growth fraction might depend on the duration of the BrdU treatment [98].

Staging

There is no general agreement for the staging of meningiomas. The usual clinical or pathomorphological (p) staging – tumor (T), (lymph) node (N), metastases (M) (TNM/pTNM) – of malignant tumors [29] is not fully applicable to meningiomas. Due to the lack of intracranial lymph vessels the N/pN classification is not possible. Also, metastases for the application of the M/pM classification are rare manifestations of hemangiopericytic, papillary, and other anaplastic meningiomas. Therefore, only other criteria such as special growth patterns may be used for a staging attempt.

Special Growth Patterns. Intraventricular meningiomas (Fig. 19.9) are most common in the trigone of the lateral ventricle but may also be found in the third ventricle [17]. Intraventricular meningiomas of the fourth ventricle are extremely rare (reviewed in [63]). All histological subtypes may occur, possibly with a certain prevalence for the fibrous subtype [27]. Anaplastic intraventricular meningiomas have been reported only twice [43, 88] but are not really rare according to my experience.

The en plaque meningioma shows another special growth pattern. Especially lateral sphenoid wing meningiomas of limited thickness display a propensity for growth along the planes of the meninges and, in some cases, occupy a considerable area (Fig. 19.10a). Spinal en plaque meningiomas in which the tumor forms a diffuse collarlike mass around the spinal cord are very rare [87].

Ectopic meningiomas may occur primarily in extracranial or extraspinal regions. Possibilities for the formation of ectopic meningiomas comprise direct extension of an intracranial lesion, origin from arachnoidal cells within the sheaths of cranial nerves, origin from embryonic nests of arachnoidal cells, and distant metastasis from an intracranial or intraspinal meningioma. Meningiomas in the orbit [16, 24] arise from the arachnoidal sheath of the intraorbital portion of the optic nerve. Primary meningiomas of the paranasal sinuses [30] may arise from arachnoidal rests left behind during embryonic development. Meningiomas of the outer surface of the skull, skin, and neck [25, 75, 91] may be explained by the anomalous presence of arachnoidal cells along the lines of fusion of the embryonic skull and spine [90]. Four cases of ectopic pulmonary meningiomas have been reviewed by Strimlan et al. [89]. All reported cases were benign tumors in asymptomatic female patients. The etiology is unknown, although several theories have been proposed by Chumas and Lorelle [14].

Pulmonary metastases from intracranial [70, 96] and intraspinal [21] meningiomas are extremely rare. Neither histological pattern, local aggressiveness, size, nor location of the tumor can be used to predict which tumors will metastasize. Except for the hemangiopericytic subtype (with a greater frequency) fewer than 1/1000 meningiomas metastasize. Som et al. [86] reviewed 113 metastasizing meningiomas reported in the literature, of which 69 did not belong to the hemangiopericytic subtype. Even histologically and cytologically benign meningiomas with well-differentiated "benign" metastases may occur [61].

In contrast, recurrences may not always be caused by anaplastic behavior of the tumor but by incomplete surgical resection. Melamed et al. [57] found a recurrence rate of 29% within 7–17 years after surgery in a series of 126 histologically entirely benign meningiomas.

In cases of type II neurofibromatosis, among other lesions, multiple cranial and spinal meningio-

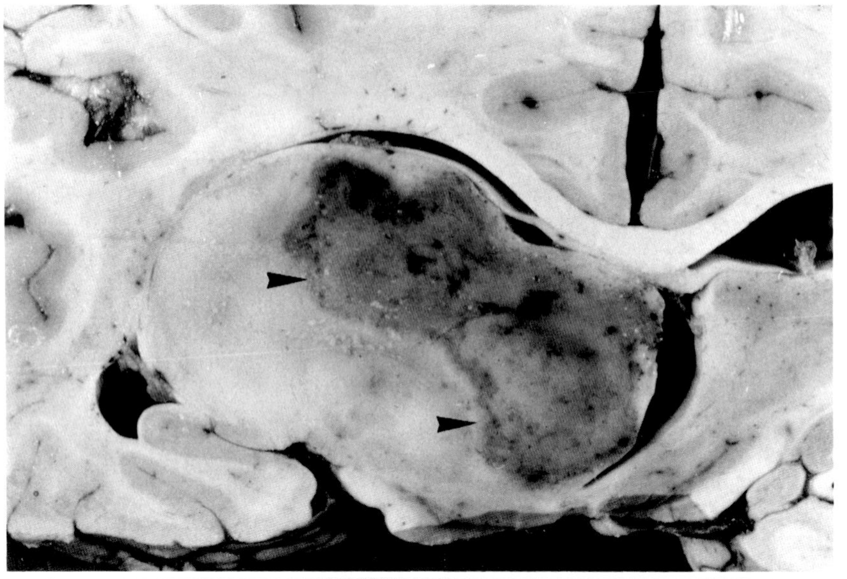

a

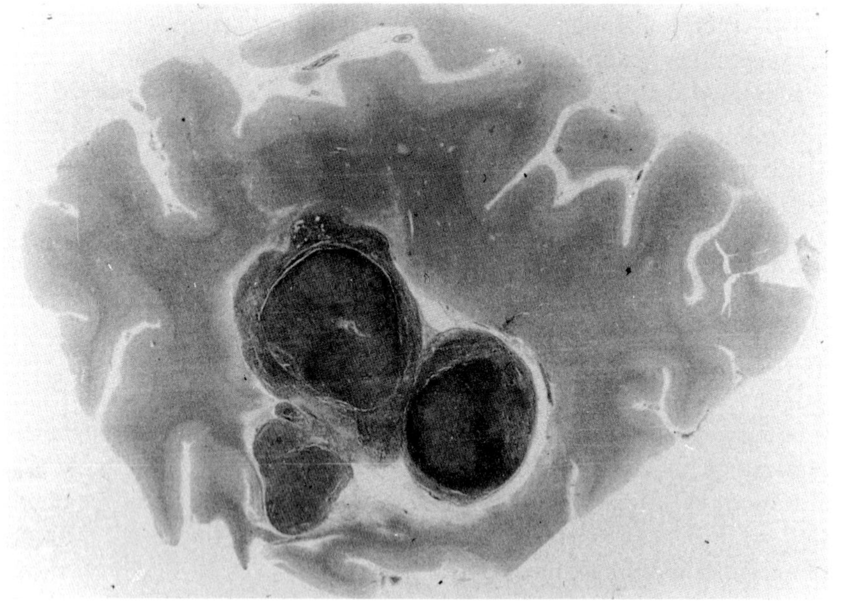

b

Fig. 19.9. **a** Intraventricular anaplastic meningioma with a large necrosis (*arrowheads*). **b** Intraventricular meningioma, incidental autopsy finding of a benign transitional meningioma (HE, large section)

Fig. 19.10. **a** Meningioma en plaque (*arrowhead*) of the sphenoid wing (Van Gieson, large section). **b** Invasive growth of a transitional meningioma into the bone of the skull (Van Gieson, ×60). **c** Invasive growth of an anaplastic meningioma into the underlying brain (HE, ×60)

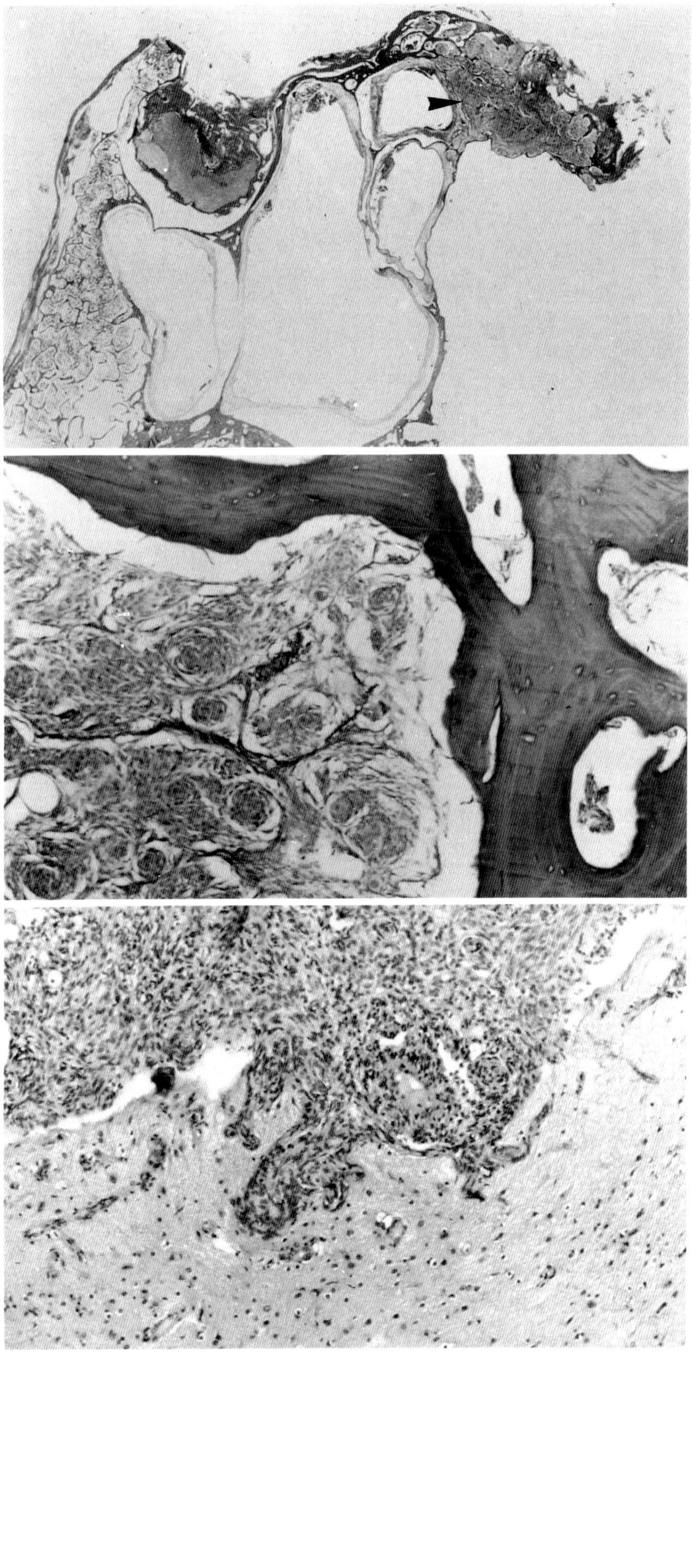

a

b

c

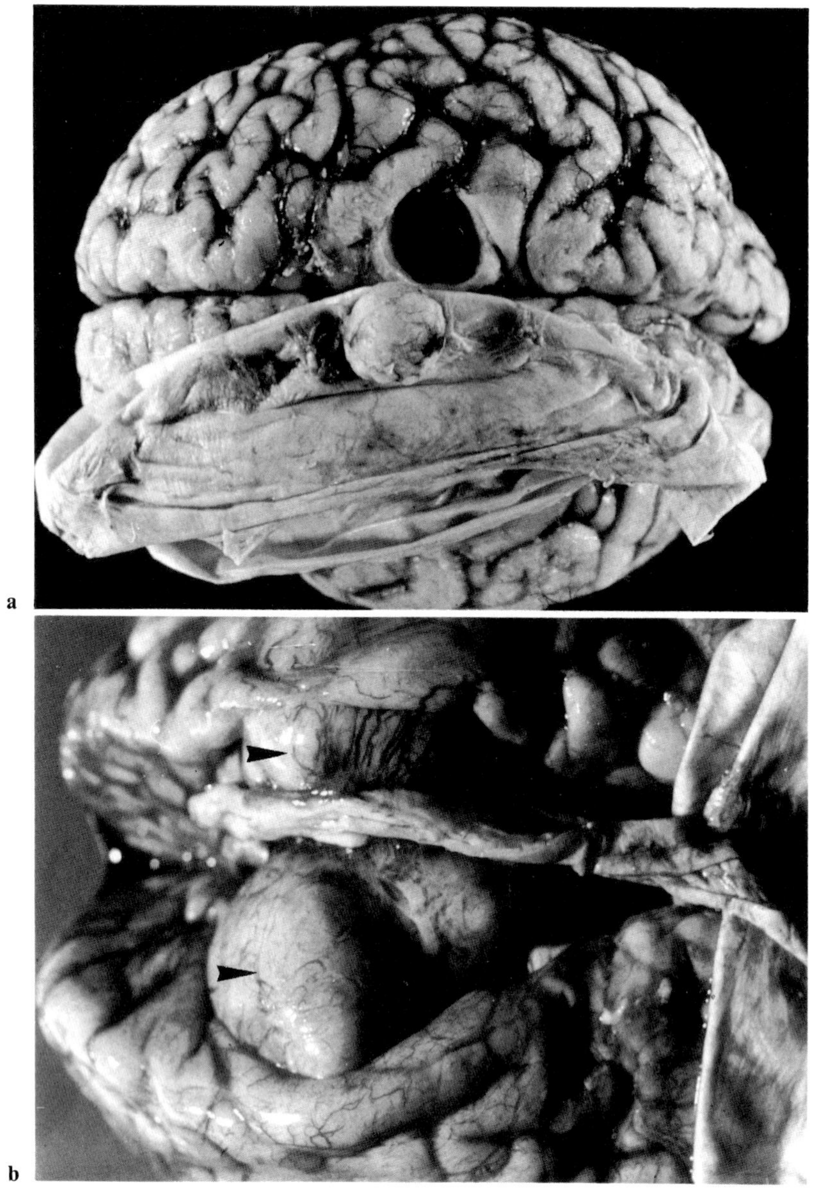

Fig. 19.11. **a** Compression atrophy of the brain cortex caused by a parasagittal meningioma. **b** Extreme intracranial expansion with increased intracranial pressure caused by a large bilateral meningioma (*arrowheads*) of the falx durae matris

mas may occur. Also, the choroid plexuses appear to be involved with unusual frequency in this meningiomatosis.

Meningiomas and Surrounding Tissue. The meningioma en plaque is often associated with a hyperostosis of the sphenoid ridge. The hyperostosis may, in some cases, be disproportionately greater than the relatively small underlying intracranial tumor [18, 41].

There may also be an invasive growth of meningiomas into the adjacent dura mater, bone, or even extraosseous soft tissue (Fig. 19.10b) which is not by itself regarded as a sign of malignancy. An invasion of the underlying brain tissue (Fig. 19.10c) is to be seen as a worrisome feature.

In brain tissue adjacent to meningiomas a compression atrophy (Fig. 19.11 a) with a certain reac-

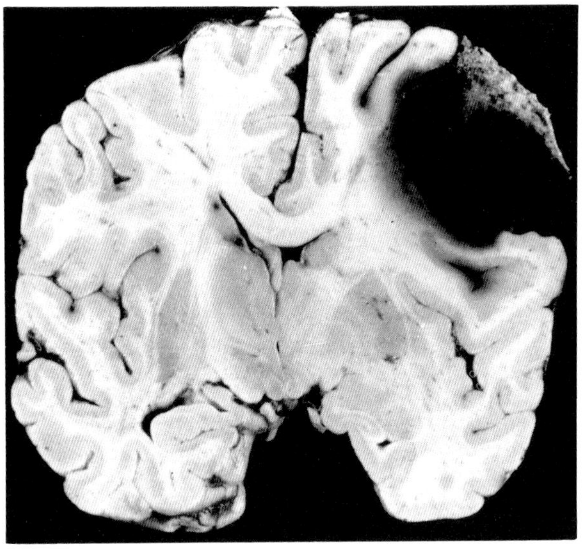

Fig. 19.12. Angiomatous meningioma with a large bleeding provoking increased intracranial pressure. Note the displaced midline of the brain

Table 19.3. Revised WHO Classification of meningiomas

Meningioma
meningothelial (syncytial)
transitional/mixed
fibrous (fibroblastic)
psammomatous
angiomatous
microcystic
secretory
clear cell
chordoid
lymphoplasmacyte-rich
metaplastic variants (xanthomatous, myxoid, osseous, cartilagineous etc.)
Atypical meningioma
Papillary meningioma
Anaplastic (malignant) meningioma

tive astrocytosis can be seen. A perifocal edema may occur, caused by an extracerebral and ensuing cerebral vascular compression [26]. Large meningiomas may provoke an increased intracranial pressure (Fig. 19.11 b).

Angiomatous meningiomas may cause a bleeding, which can also lead to an increased intracranial pressure (Fig. 19.12).

Addendum in Proof

A Working Group of the World Health Organization (WHO) has been established in order to revise the histological classification of brain tumors [101]. This revision will be published in near future and comprises as new entities many of the special meningioma subtypes described in this chapter (Table 19.3). On the other hand, the hemangiopericytoma will be listed as mesenchymal, non-meningothelial tumor which certainly is justified regarding the many differences between this entity and "typical" meningiomas. The hemangioblastoma will be listed as tumor of uncertain origin, a prudent decision considering its occurrence as hemangioblastic meningioma and as Lindau tumor. A comment must be given on the newly introduced distinction between atypical and anaplastic meningiomas. Whereas anaplastic meningiomas reveal all signs of malignancy as described above, atypical meningiomas are meningiomas with an in general slightly or moderately increased mitotic rate and a tendency to recurrence. Cellular polymorphism (atypia) may be observed but is not obligatory. Atypical meningiomas must not behave malignant (i.e. sarcoma-like as anaplastic meningiomas) but a tight follow-up of the patients is recommendable.

References

1. Ahyai A, Spaar FW (1987) DNA and prognosis of meningiomas: a comparative cytological and fluorescence-cytophotometrical study of 71 tumors. Acta Neurochir (Wien) 87:119–128
2. Ahyai A, Zimmermann A, Spaar FW (1983) Flow fluorescence cytometry of deoxyribonucleic acid in meningiomas: studies on surgically removed tumor specimens compared with their cells in primary tissue cultures. Surg Neurol 20:194–205
3. Al Saadi A, Latimer F, Madercic M, Robbins T (1987) Cytogenetic studies of human brain tumors and their clinical significance. II. Meningioma. Cancer Genet Cytogenet 26:127–141
4. Alguacil-Garcia A, Pettigrew NW, Sima AAF (1986) Secretory meningioma. A distinct subtype of meningioma. Am J Surg Pathol 10:102–111
5. Andres KH (1967) Über die Feinstruktur der Arachnoidea und Dura mater von Mammalia. Z Zellforsch 79:272–295
6. Arinami T, Kondo I, Hamaguchi H, Nakajima S (1986) Multifocal meningiomas in a patient with a constitutional ring chromosome 22. J Med Genet 23:178–180

7. Banerjee AK, Blackwood W (1971) A subfrontal tumour with the features of plasmocytoma and meningioma. Acta Neuropathol (Berl) 18:84–88
8. Bickerstaff ER, Small JM, Guest IA (1958) The relapsing course of certain meningiomas in relation to pregnancy and menstruation. J Neurol Neurosurg Psychiatry 121:89–91
9. Bishop JM (1983) Cellular oncogenes and retroviruses. Annu Rev Biochem 52:301–354
10. Bolger GB, Stamberg J, Kirsch IR, Hollis GF, Schwarz DF, Thomas GH (1985) Chromosome translocation t (14; 22) and oncogene (c-sis) variant in a pedigree with familial meningioma. N Engl J Med 312:564–567
11. Borges LF (1986) Laminin immunostaining predicts biological behavior of meningiomas (Poster). 55th Annual Meeting of the American Association of Neurological Surgeons, Denver
12. Burger PC, Shibata T, Kleihues P (1986) The use of the monoclonal antibody Ki-67 in the identification of proliferating cells: application to surgical neuropathology. Am J Surg Pathol 10:611–617
13. Cho KG, Hoshino T, Nagashima T, Murovic JA, Wilson CB (1986) Prediction of tumor doubling time in recurrent meningiomas. Cell kinetics studies with bromodeoxyuridine labeling. J Neurosurg 65:790–794
14. Chumas CJ, Lorelle CA (1982) Pulmonary meningioma: a light-electron-microscopic study. Am J Surg Pathol 6:795–801
15. Churg A (1985) Immunohistochemical staining for vimentin and keratin in malignant mesothelioma. Am J Surg Pathol 9:360–365
16. Crain WM, Gozela LJ (1949) Intraorbital meningiomas. Am J Ophthalmol 32:1663–1680
17. Criscuolo GR, Symon L (1986) Intraventricular meningioma. A review of 10 cases of the National Hospital, Queen Square (1974–1985) with reference to the literature. Acta Neurochir (Wien) 83:83–91
18. Cushing H (1922) The cranial hyperostoses produced by meningeal endotheliomas. Arch Neurol Psychiatr 8:139–154
19. Cushing H, Eisenhardt L (1938) Meningiomas. Their classification, regional behaviour, life history, and surgical end results. Thomas, Springfield
20. Dahmen HG (1979) Studies of mucous substances in myxomatous meningiomas. Acta Neuropathol (Berl) 48:235–237
21. Dastur KJ, Reza Raji M, Smith WI Jr (1984) Pulmonary metastasis from intraspinal meningioma. Am J Neuroradiol 5:483–484
22. Fortuna A, Ferrante L, Acqui M, Guglielmi G, Mastronardi L (1988) Cystic meningiomas. Acta Neurochir (Wien) 90:23–30
23. Frederiksen P, Reske-Nielsen E, Bichel P (1979) DNA content of meningiomas. Acta Neuropathol (Berl) 46:65–68
24. Gabibov GA, Blinkov SM, Tcherekayev VA (1988) The management of optic nerve meningiomas and gliomas. J Neurosurg 68:889–893
25. Geoffray A, Lee YY, Jing BS, Wallace S (1983) Extracranial meningiomas of the head and neck. AJNR 5:599–604
26. Ginsbourg M, Le Beau J (1979) Histoenzymatic and permeability changes in human brain adjacent to meningioma. J Neuropathol Exp Neurol 38:47–56
27. Guidetti B, Delfini R, Gagliardi FM, Vagnozzi R (1985) Meningiomas of the lateral ventricles. Clinical, neuroradiologic, and surgical considerations in 19 cases. Surg Neurol 24:364–370
28. Harrison JD, Rose PE (1985) Myxoid meningioma: histochemistry and electron microscopy. Acta Neuropathol (Berl) 68:80–82
29. Hermanek P, Sobin LH (1987) TNM classification of malignant tumours, 4th edn. International Union Against Cancer, Geneva
30. Ho KL (1980) Primary meningioma of the nasal cavity and paranasal sinuses. Cancer 46:1442–1447
31. Holden J, Dolman CL, Churg A (1987) Immunohistochemistry of meningiomas including the angioblastic type. J Neuropathol Exp Neurol 46:50–56
32. Hossmann KA, Zülch KJ (1966) Die spinalen psammomatösen Meningeome der Frau. Neurochirurgia (Stuttg) 9:106–113
33. Ironside JW, Battersby RDE, Lawry J, Loomes RS, Day CA, Timperley WR (1987) DNA in meningioma tissues and explant cell cultures. A flow cytometric study with clinicopathological correlates. J Neurosurg 66:588–594
34. Iwaki T, Takeshita I, Fukui M, Kitamura K (1987) Cell kinetics of the malignant evolution of meningothelial meningioma. Acta Neuropathol (Berl) 74:243–247
35. Iwaki T, Fukui M, Takeshita I, Tsuneyoshi M, Tateishi J (1988) Hemangiopericytoma of the meninges: a clinicopathologic and immunohistochemical study. Clin Neuropathol 7:93–99
36. Katsuyama J, Papenhausen PP, Herz F, Gazivoda P, Hirano A, Koss LG (1986) Chromosome abnormalities in meningiomas. Cancer Genet Cytogenet 22:63–68
37. Kawano H, Hayashi M, Kabuto M, Kobayashi H, Handa Y, Kubota T, Satoh K (1988) An immunohistochemical and ultrastructural study of cultured intracranial hemangiopericytoma. Clin Neuropathol 7:105–110
38. Kendall B, Reider-Grosswasser I, Valentine A (1983) Diagnosis of masses presenting within the ventricles on computed tomography. Neuroradiology 25:11–22
39. Kepes JJ (1982) Meningiomas. Biology, pathology, and differential diagnosis. Year Book Medical Publishers, Chicago
40. Kepes JJ (1986) Presidential address: the histopathology of meningiomas. A reflection of origins and expected behaviour. J Neuropathol Exp Neurol 45:95–107
41. Kim SK, Rogers LF, Goldblatt D (1987) CT features of hyperostosing meningioma en plaque. AJNR 8: 853–859
42. Kleinert R, Radner H (1987) Lectin binding in meningiomas. Neuropathol Applied Neurobiol 13:263–272
43. Kleinschmidt-DeMasters BK, Avakian JJ (1985) Wallenberg syndrome caused by CSF metastasis from malignant intraventricular meningioma. Clin Neuropathol 4:214–219
44. Knudson AG (1985) Hereditary cancer, oncogenes, and antioncogenes. Cancer Res 45:1437–1443

45. Laerum OD, Farsund T (1981) Clinical application of flow cytometry: a review. Cytometry 2:1–13
46. LaRocca PJ, Rheinwald JG (1984) Coexpression of simple epithelial keratins and vimentin by human mesothelium and mesothelioma in vivo and in culture. Cancer Res 44:2991–2999
47. Lehmann J, Krug H (1980) Flow-through fluorocytophotometry of different brain tumours. Acta Neuropathol (Berl) 49:123–132
48. Lesch KP, Gross S (1987) Estrogen receptor immunoreactivity in meningiomas. Comparison with the binding activity of estrogen, progesterone, and androgen receptors. J Neurosurg 67:237–243
49. Lesch KP, Schott W, Engl HG, Gross S, Thierauf P (1987) Gonadal steroid receptors in meningiomas. J Neurol 234:328–333
50. Lopez-Gines C, Piquer J, Cerda-Nicolas M, Barcia-Salorio J, Barcia-Marino C (1989) Meningiomas: karyotypes and histological pattern. Clin Neuropathol 8:130–133
51. Mark J (1977) Chromosomal abnormalities and their specifity in human neoplasms: an assessment of recent observations by banding technique. Adv Cancer Res 74:165–170
52. Markwalder TM, Zava DT, Goldhirsch A (1983) Estrogen and progesterone receptors in relation to clinical and pathological features. Surg Neurol 20:42–47
53. Markwalder TM, Waelti E, König MP (1987) Endocrine manipulation of meningiomas with medroxyprogesterone acetate. Effect of MPA on receptor status of meningioma cytosols. Surg Neurol 28:3–9
54. Markwalder TM, Gerber HA, Waelti E, Schaffner T, Markwalder RV (1988) Hormonetherapy of meningiomas with medroxyoprogeserone acetate. Immunohistochemical demonstration of the effect of medroxyprogesterone acetate on growth fractions of meningioma cells using the monoclonal antibody Ki-67. Surg Neurol 30:97–101
55. Martuza RL, Seizinger BR, Jacoby LB, Rouleau GA, Gusella JF (1988) The molecular biology of human glial tumors. TINS 11:22–27
56. McDonald JD, Dohrmann GJ (1988) Molecular biology of brain tumors. Neurosurgery 23:537–544
57. Melamed S, Sahar A, Beller AJ (1979) The recurrence of intracranial meningiomas. Neurochirurgia (Stuttg) 22:47–51
58. Mendiratta SS, Rosenblum JA, Strobos RJ (1967) Congenital meningioma. Neurology (Minneap) 17: 914–918
59. Mennel HD, Zinngrebe J, Berweiler-Nippert U, Lorenz H (1988) Meningiomas: histogenesis and classification. A comparative morphological study. Zentralbl Allg Pathol 134:27–40
60. Merten DF, Gooding CA, Newton TH, Malamud N (1974) Meningiomas in childhood and adolescence. J Pediatr 84:696–700
61. Miller CD, Ojemann RG, Proppe KH, McGinnis BD, Grillo HC (1985) Benign metastasizing meningioma. Case report. J Neurosurg 62:763–766
62. Moss TH (1987) Immunohistochemical characteristics of haemangiopericytic meningiomas: comparison with typical meningiomas, haemangioblastomas and haemangiopericytomas from extracranial sites. Neuropathol Appl Neurobiol 13:467–480
63. Nagata K, Basugi N, Sasaki T, Hashimoto K, Manaka S, Takakura K (1988) Intraventricular meningioma of the fourth ventricle. Case report. Neurol Med Chir 28:86–90
64. Nagle RB, McDaniel KM, Clark VA, Payne CM (1983) The use of anti-keratin antibodies in the diagnosis of human tumours. Am J Clin Pathol 79:458–466
65. Nakamura M, Inoue HK, Ono N, Kunimine H, Tamada J (1987) Analysis of hemangiopericytic meningiomas by immunohistochemistry, electron microscopy and cell culture. J Neuropathol Exp Neurol 46:57–71
66. Nakasu S, Hirano A, Shimura T, Llena JF (1987) Incidental meningiomas in autopsy study. Surg Neurol 27:319–322
67. Namer IJ, Pamir MN, Benli K, Saglam S, Erbengi A (1987) Spinal meningiomas. Neurochirurgia (Stuttg) 30:11–15
68. Olson JJ, Beck DW, Schlechte JA, Loh PM (1987) Effect of the antiprogesterone RU-38486 on meningioma implanted into nude mice. J Neurosurg 66:584–587
69. Osborn M (1983) Intermediate filaments as histological markers: an overview. J Invest Dermatol [Suppl] 81:104–109
70. Peck AG, Dedrick CG, Taft PD (1976) Pulmonary metastases from intracerebral meningioma: diagnosis by percutaneous needle aspiration biopsy. AJR 126: 419–422
71. Poisson M, Pertuiset BF, Hauw JJ (1983) Steroid hormone receptors in human meningiomas, gliomas and brain metastases. J Neurooncol 1:179–189
72. Poulsgård L, Rønne M, Schrøder HD (1989) Cytogenetic studies of 19 meningiomas and their clinical significance. I. Anticancer Res 9:109–112
73. Rand CW, Andler M (1950) Tumors of the brain complicating pregnancy. Arch Neurol Psychiatry 163:1–42
74. Rausing A, Ybo W, Stenflo J (1970) Intracranial meningioma. A population study of ten years. Acta Neurol Scand 46:102–110
75. Rose WS, Makhija MC, Sattenspiel S (1980) Meningioma presenting as tumor in the neck. AJR 134: 1070–1072
76. Rossi ML, Cruz Sanchez F, Hughes JT, Esiri MM, Coakham HB (1988) Immunocytochemical study of the cellular immune response in meningiomas. J Clin Pathol 41:314–319
77. Rubinstein LJ (1972) Tumors of the central nervous system. Armed Forces Institute of Pathology, Washington, pp 169–190 (Atlas of tumor pathology, 2nd ser, fasc 6)
78. Rubenstein LJ (1982) Tumors of the central nervous system. Armed Forces Institute of Pathology, Washington, pp 9–13 (Atlas of tumor pathology, 2nd ser, fasc 6, suppl)
79. Rutherford GS, Marus G (1987) Microcystic meningiomas. Clin Neuropathol 6:143–148
80. Sasaki S, Nakagawa K, Kimura H, Ohue S (1987) Intracranial meningiomas in infancy. Surg Neurol 28:51–57

81. Schmidek HH (1987) The molecular genetics of nervous system tumors. J Neurosurg 67:1–16
82. Schober R, Himuro H, Wechsler W (1988) Cystic changes and vascular permeability in meningiomas. Clin Neuropathol 7:16–21
83. Schoenberg BS, Christine BW, Whisnant JP (1975) Nervous system neoplasms and primary malignancies of other sites: the unique association between meningiomas and breast cancer. Neurology (Minneap) 25:705–712
84. Schwechheimer K, Kartenbeck J, Moll R, Franke WW (1984) Vimentin filament-desmosome cytoskeleton of diverse types of human meningiomas. A distinctive diagnostic feature. Lab Invest 51:584–591
85. Seizinger BR, de la Monte S, Atkins L, Gusella JF, Martuza RL (1987) Molecular genetic approach to human meningioma: loss of genes on chromosome 22. Proc Natl Acad Sci USA 84:5419–5423
86. Som PM, Sacher M, Strenger SW, Biller HF, Malis LI (1986) "Benign" metastasizing meningiomas. AJNR 8:127–130
87. Stechison MT, Tasker RR, Wortzman G (1987) Spinal meningioma en plaque. Report of two cases. J Neurosurg 67:452–455
88. Strenger SW, Huang YP, Sachdev VP (1987) Malignant meningioma within the third ventricle: a case report. Neurosurgery 20:465–468
89. Strimlan CV, Golembiewski RS, Celko DA, Fino GF (1988) Primary pulmonary meningioma. Surg Neurol 29:410–413
90. Suzuki H, Gilbert EF, Zimmerman B (1967) Primary extracranial meningioma. Arch Pathol 84:202–206
91. Tampieri D, Pokrupa R, Melanson D, Ethier R (1987) Primary ectopic meningioma of the neck. J Comput Assist Tomogr 11:1054–1056
92. Terpe HJ, Kasper M, Martin H, Lehmann J (1988) Nachweis von Zytokeratin in Zellen der Arachnoidea und in Meningiomen. Zentralbl Allg Pathol 134: 259–264
93. Van Landegem W, Vakaet A, de Paepe A, Verschraegen-Spae MR (1988) Familial meningioma. Case report with cytogenetic study. Clin Neurol Neurosurg 90:61–63
94. Walker AE, Robins M, Weinfeld FD (1985) Epidemiology of brain tumors: the national survery of intracranial neoplasms. Neurology 35:219–226
95. Weber T, Liebert UG, Wechsler W (1983) Immunocytochemical identification of factor VIII and *Ulex europaeus* type I lectin binding in endothelial cells in human vascular meningiomas (Abstr). Acta Neurol Scand 68:198
96. Wende S, Bohl J, Schubert R, Schulz V (1983) Lung metastasis of a meningioma. Neuroradiology 24: 287–291
97. Wood MW, White RJ, Kernohan JW (1957) One hundred intracranial meningiomas found incidentally at necropsy. J Neuropathol Exp Neurol 16:337–340
98. Yoshii Y, Maki Y, Tsuboi K, Tomono Y, Nakagawa K, Hoshino T (1986) Estimation of growth fraction with bromodeoxyuridine in human central nervous system tumors. J Neurosurg 65:659–663
99. Yung WKA, Borit A, Dahl D, Wang E (1984) Keratin and vimentin in meningiomas (Abstr). J Neuropathol Exp Neurol 43:299
100. Zang KD (1982) Cytological and cytogenetical studies on human meningioma. Cancer Genet Cytogenet 6:249–274
101. Zülch KJ (ed) (1979) Histological typing of tumours of the central nervous system. World Health Organization, Geneva (International histological classification of tumours, no 21)
102. Zülch KJ (1986) Brain tumors. Their biology and pathology. Springer, Berlin Heidelberg New York
103. Zülch KJ, Schmid EE (1955) Über das Ependymom, den Seitenventrikel und Foramen Monroi. Arch Psychiatr Zentralbl Neurol 193:214–228

Subject Index